That's Good Grease

That's
Good
Grease

And Other Surprising
Compliments
About Hospice

Rick Schneider

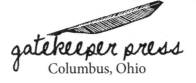
gatekeeper press
Columbus, Ohio

That's Good Grease: And Other Surprising Compliments about Hospice

Published by Gatekeeper Press
3971 Hoover Rd. Suite 77
Columbus, OH 43123-2839
www.GatekeeperPress.com

ISBN: 9781619847873
eISBN: 9781619847866

Printed in the United States of America

To James T. (Jim) Schneider

TABLE OF CONTENTS

ACKNOWLEDGEMENTS 11

INTRODUCTION 15

~ That's Good Grease ~ 17

~ Where I Volunteer ~ 21

~ A Few Hospice Myths~ 23

~ When Was Hospice Invented? ~ 27

~ Now A Person ~ 29

~ Total Comfort ~ 31

~ A Familiar Word ~ 35

~ Celebrate Independence ~ 39

~ Celebrate the Fourth ~ 41

~ Check Engine Light ~ 43

~ Communicating Doesn't Just Mean Talking ~ 45

~ Don't be Dreary ~ 49

~ Enjoy the end of life? ~ 51

~ Father's Day Gift ~ 53

~ Financial Relief ~ 55

~ Ginger Bread Cupcakes with Green Icing ~ 57

~ Gratitude List ~ 59

~ Have You Turned Around? ~ 61

~Hospice is Easy ~ 63

~ Unique, Just Like the Others ~ 65

~ How the Story Ends ~ 69

~ Hospice Chaplains Are Important ~ 71

~ Let's Live a Little ~ 75

~ Should We Call? ~ 77

~ Acceptance ~ 81

~ Definitely Not a Mistake ~ 85

~ The Cavalry is Here ~ 87

~ Back in control ~ 89

~ The Old Mattress ~ 91

~ The Medicine was Taken Away ~ 93

~ This Just Can't be Happening ~ 95

~ Volunteers ~ 97

~ We Have Time ~ 99

~ We Help Remove Fear ~ 101

~ It's Life Expectancy, Not Disease ~ 103

~ You Can't Call Too Soon ~ 105

~ Palliative Care ~ 107

~ F.A.S.T. Scale ~...111

~ What Kind of a Place is Hospice? ~.....................................115

~ Can't Beat the Price ~ 117

~ Making St. Peter Wait ~..121

~ Which Doctor ~ 123

~ You Won't be Swept Away ~ 125

~ Your Bucket List ~ 127

~ A Deer for the Deer Hunter ~ 131

~ A Mother's Love ~ 133

~ Thoughtful, Committed People ~ 137

~ A Wonderful Fall Wedding ~ 141

~ Basic Nursing ~ 143

~ Bob's Unforgettable Dance ~ 145

~ Celebrate the Lasts ~...147

~ This Night Was Different ~ 149

~ Dogs Just Know ~..151

~ Cats May Not Seem Interested ~...153

~ Graduating from Hospice ~..155

~ It is of Absolute Importance ~...157

~ All in the Family ~ 159

~ Everyone Affected ~..161

~ Hospice Nurse ~ 163

~ Importance of Food ~...165

~ The Family's Perspective ~ 169

~ Good-byes are Necessary ~..173

~ Hospice is a Life Sentence ~...175

~ Look at All Sides ~ 177

~ I C U or the Kitchen? ~ 181

~ It's the Little Things ~ 183

~ Lonely Patient ~ 185
~ Massage Therapy ~ 187
~ A Lot of Good People ~ 189
~ The Final Vow ~ 193
~ From Music to Spirituality ~ 195
~ One Last Fair Cookie ~ 197
~ Pepper ~ 199
 ~ Respite ~ 201
~ Security Prayer ~ 203
~ Subtle Spirituality ~ 205
~ Someone Understands ~ 209
~ The Air Mattress ~ 211
~ The Final Act of Love ~ 213
~ Yes, The Little Things ~ 215
~ Why Won't They Eat ~ 217
~ I'll Wear This One ~ 221
~ All of This is For You ~ 227
~ Time ~ 229
~ What a Day for a Picnic ~ 231
~ Why Have Doctors on Staff? ~ 233
~ When Most Needed ~ 237
~ Ernie and I ~ 239
~ He Had Purpose ~ 241
~ Back Into Perspective ~ 243
~ They do Grieve ~ 245
~ Graduations ~ 247
~ I Love the Fair ~ 251
~ Is it That Time Already? ~ 253
~ One Card Twice ~ 257
~ One New Year's Resolution ~ 259
~ Oscar ~ 261
~ People Are the Important Part ~ 263
~ People Know We Care ~ 267
~ She Left as She Came ~ 269
~ Single Bells ~ 271
~ Support Afterwards ~ 273

~ Survivors of a Suicide Death ~ 277

~ What about the Young People? ~ 279

~ Attention and Respect ~..281

~ Avoid Clichés Like the Plague ~...283

~ Cab Ride to Hospice ~...285

~ Chester Consoling ~ 289

~ Everyday War Stories ~ 291

~ We Don't Know Them All ~ 293

~ Veteran's Day ~...297

~Even a Little Fawn ~ 299

~ Compassionate, Creative People ~...301

~ Oh, I Don't Want to Hear About That ~...303

~ Normal, Everyday People ~ **305**

~ Pet Therapy ~...309

~ Dogs Feel it Too ~ 311

~ Thanks, Dad ~ 313

~ Thanksgiving ~ 315

~ Volunteers are Necessary ~ 317

~ What Needs Doing ~ 321

~ What is it like to be a Hospice Patient-Contact Volunteer? ~.........323

~ Endings to Beginnings ~ 327

~ Without Charging a Penny ~..329

~ Why Volunteer? ~ 331

~ Just A Simple Pinning ~ 333

~ Darling, We Made It ~..337

~ Laughing Matters ~..339

~ Life's Two Big Events ~ 343

~ Put Your Life Back in Order ~ 345

~ She Did it Again ~..347

~ Still a Salesman ~ 349

~ Volunteer There? ~...353

~ Where'd Everyone Go? ~ 357

~ Why Not Tell Them Now ~...359

ACKNOWLEDGEMENTS

I THANK MY WIFE, Vickie, for her patience as I pursued my passion of being available to those on hospice service. She was my subconscious reason for becoming a hospice volunteer in the first place. Her forty-year nursing career was spent in nursing homes. She always chose to work second shift, allowing for more direct patient care. There were times when she'd call me near the end of her shift, around 11:30 p.m., and I knew what she'd say. One of the nursing home residents was actively dying and she was going to stay with them.

Why would she stay? There were several reasons for that. Maybe the person had no surviving family, but more often it was because the family contact said thanks for calling, just "Let me know when she's gone." Vickie said that she just couldn't let the person die alone, so she'd stay with them until they died or until first shift came in to relieve her. She never considered asking to be paid for those hours.

In September of 1996, my siblings had called a family meeting at Mom's bedside. Her health was declining and she had signed Advanced Directives years before stating that she wanted no heroic measures done. While there, Vickie noticed Mom's signs of imminent death and told us that we should each take the time, now, to say our good-byes. I never knew that there were indicators of natural death, but my wife was right; Mom was gone within three hours. What a blessing it was to have the opportunity to thank her for all her sacrifices for me. As a side note, after we finished saying our good-byes Vickie brushed Mom's hair and put make-up on her so she would, "Look good for Jesus." Hearing that, Mom gave us her last, albeit faint, smile.

In addition to Vickie, there are others who helped me along the way. In particular, I must thank Denise Bauer, R.N., for making this book possible. As first Clinical Director, then CEO of FairHoPe

Hospice and Palliative Care, Inc. she was a true servant of the people on service and their families. She gave her staff and volunteers the confidence to do what they thought the person on service needed. Her presence created the atmosphere of love and compassion that FairHoPe was noted for. Denise epitomized the truth that you don't raise morale in an organization; it starts at the top and filters down.

Thank you to my long-time coworker and mentor, Chaplain Karl Hartmann. Karl was FairHoPe's only chaplain for many years, and is still a part time chaplain. I assisted Karl with many grief support groups and memorial services. He showed me that values are caught, not taught. Karl demonstrated the essence of God's love by joyfully accepting everyone who came on hospice service, regardless of belief system, background, or appearance.

Thank you to Susan Foglesong, who shared an office with me for years and was always there to make insightful suggestions about my writing, pull me out of computer trouble, or keep me out of it in the first place.

Thanks to Twylia Summers, FairHoPe's Director of Volunteers, who has been my mentor, fellow volunteer, coworker, adviser, and friend. Over the years, Twylia has given me many writing ideas.

Thank you to Tammy Drobina, my contact at the Fairfield Towne Crier newspaper, whose input and encouragement has been invaluable. Deb Tobin, Editor of the Logan Daily News, more or less insisted that I submit a long article every two weeks, although she wanted a weekly article. Also, my thanks to Rebecca Hedges, at the Logan Daily, for her frequent words of encouragement.

I must also thank my daughter, Lindsey Schneider, who proofed my writing, helped to determine article themes, and occasionally went with me to visit my hospice patients and to attend hospice-sponsored events. Thanks to The Pickering House Kitchen Manager, Linda Foglesong, who uses the common thread of food to gain access to our patients' hearts. Examples of her empathy and love are spread throughout this book.

Thank you to Tracey Miller, FairHoPe Hospice's Children's Grief Coordinator, for her input regarding children's grief. She taught me that even when the "children" had achieved adulthood, the parent-child relationship is always there. Thank you to social worker Ernie Doling – we had quite a few adventures together at FairHoPe. He is a part of a story or two in the book. Thank you to Tammie Morris-Koetz, R.N., for her encouragement and support of my writing by posting my stories on social media.

I also owe a special debt of gratitude to Kristin Glasure who was my instructor during volunteer training and my first supervisor as patient care volunteer back in early 1997. Even as of this writing, Kristin, currently our Director of Social Services, is always available to drop what she is doing and assist me.

Social Worker Naomi Colvin, who has helped patients finish knitting and sewing projects, Mary Scott R.N., Tammy Sullivan R.N., Heidi Crum R.N., Pat Disbennet and Carla Munyan, have all shared with me many ideas and thoughts about end-of-life care. Several stories contained in this book are a result of conversations with them. Over the past 20 years there have been so many others: Shelia C., Heather R., Kathy D., Sheila M., Loren H., Shelli, Kristin, Lora, Patsy, Norma, Ed V., etc.

And a special thank you to FairHoPe Hospice's wonderful volunteers, several of whom are a part of the stories included in this book. It is so difficult to get stories out of them because of their humility. They sometimes don't see anything special or noteworthy in their actions. I hear a completely different story from those who have benefitted from their selfless love.

My apologies if I forgot anyone; so many have been a part of this journey.

It has been, and still is, a pleasure to serve those who come to hospice.

INTRODUCTION

~ THAT'S GOOD GREASE ~

SEVERAL YEARS AGO, a woman was admitted to The Pickering House, FairHoPe Hospice and Palliative Care, Inc.'s in-patient facility, for end-of-life care. She had been sleeping for most of the past several days which is not an unusual occurrence as life ebbs. On this particular day, she woke up with a beautiful smile and started talking about how hungry she was. In her room when she awoke were her grown daughter and a nurse's aide. The aide asked her what she thought she might like to eat. Even though at first they thought they misunderstood her, the aide and the daughter determined that the patient wanted a "junior" bacon cheeseburger and a diet cola from a fast food restaurant.

Concerned because of the woman's inability to chew or swallow, the aide knew the request was out of the question. However, being a Pickering House staff member, she also knew that something could be done, but what? The daughter respectfully asked her mom if she would actually be able to eat such a sandwich. "No," she said, "but if I could just have a lick."

Maybe it was a coincidence but at that moment the kitchen manager, Linda, entered the room and asked the patient if she was hungry. The woman repeated her request. Linda, without flinching, said that she could fix the bacon cheeseburger made with fresh hamburger from the local butcher shop and use high grade cheese from the farmer's market. The woman was all for it, so it was settled. "One junior bacon cheeseburger with a diet cola, comin' up."

The aide went to a nearby convenience store and bought the diet cola. Soon the order of a diet cola and a bacon cheeseburger, made with high quality beef and cheese, was brought to the woman's room. The daughter was flabbergasted; she couldn't believe the effort put into a seemingly insignificant request for her mom. (Linda confided to me later that she sensed this was the woman's last supper and wasn't about to talk her out of it.)

Looking at the stacked sandwich, the woman knew she couldn't eat it but asked if she could just have a bite of the bacon. The daughter cautioned her not to choke, so Linda said she would crumble a piece into little bits. She then crushed a piece of the bacon into bits between two spoons. The aroma of the bacon from the sandwich smelled so "Sunday morning-ish." The woman asked if she could lick the bacon grease off one of the spoons, which she did.

"That's good grease!" the mother exclaimed. "Oh, that is such good grease," she softly repeated to herself as she lay back on her pillow, radiating a smile. With eyes moistening the daughter whispered, "I'll remember this moment for the rest of my life."

The aide, realizing that this was becoming a spiritual moment, gingerly drew out some diet cola from the can with an eye dropper and let a few drops fall on the woman's tongue. "Nectar of the gods," the woman said with a sigh. The look on her face was pure euphoria as she experienced the wonderful taste of what she had missed for so long. The woman's request for the bacon cheeseburger was against all medical advice and, of course, all common sense. It was, however, an absolutely essential request for someone who wanted something "one last time."

Hospice is a wonderful philosophy of care, yet no one wants to hear about it. I have been a patient-contact volunteer with FairHoPe Hospice and Palliative Care, Inc. in Lancaster, Ohio since March of 1997. I've been astounded, repeatedly, at the effect something as insignificant as bacon grease has on not only the person on service but their family. What has also astounded me is how quickly the staff of FairHoPe Hospice picks up on the little indicators that a quiet suggestion is deep down a heartfelt special request.

I believe that most hospices tend to go to great lengths to comfort those they serve. The hospice art of comforting is a holistic approach involving three areas: Physical, emotional, and spiritual. In the last stage of life, the physical arena involves mostly pain control; we really don't want to give the disease any more attention than it has already received. As a patient contact volunteer, I have witnessed how spiritual pain and emotional pain, generally ignored in the medical field, are often the cause of physical pain.

I got involved with hospice service in a roundabout way. I think it was a "God Thang" as we used to say. On a cold January Sunday in 1997, I was sitting at the kitchen table browsing through the local paper, the Lancaster Eagle Gazette, just reading the headlines and turning the pages. On one of the pages was a one-inch ad that simply stated, "Hospice Seeking Volunteers." Below the headline was the phone number to call for more information. That's all there was, no hype, no save the world, just that hospice was seeking volunteers. There was no question in my mind, I knew that I had to do it.

Over the years as a patient contact volunteer I became a witness to, and a part of, the beauty of what we do in hospice. I became aware of how all the myths of hospice were borne out of fear and contempt without investigation. FairHoPe Hospice was doing so many wonderful things for those on our service, yet no one wanted to hear about it. Over time, I started keeping short notes about some of what I experienced as a volunteer. Eventually those notes became essays and I submitted a few Letters to the Editor in the local paper, or as articles in the Ohio Hospice and Palliative Care Organization's quarterly publication, "*In Touch*," (O.H.P.C.O. is now LeadingAge Ohio).

The easiest way for me to dispel the misconceptions of what we do is by gently explaining through FairHoPe's staff and my own experiences, how much can be done for a person during the last stage of life. The general public tells me that they are surprised at how much of hospice compassion does not involve medicine.

In this book, I dispel some of the myths of hospice through what I have experienced at FairHoPe Hospice and Palliative Care, Inc. as a patient contact volunteer. It's important to remember that each hospice is unique and performs their service in the manner they feel is best. Each hospice, to be Medicare certified, must adhere to the government's guidelines. How they follow the guidelines is it up to each individual hospice.

It's also important to understand that there are basically two types of hospice organizations: Not-For-Profit hospices, such as mine, and For-Profit hospices. Both types perform a wonderful service to their communities. The Not-For-Profit hospices ordinarily require financial assistance through fundraisers and donations. For those who contribute, know that it's money well spent.

For the woman I described above, such a simple pleasure as the taste of bacon was so easy to provide and displayed the common-sense attitude of hospice staff in general. At the end of her life, this woman did not have to be concerned with, "It's not good for you." The staff's only concern was how to make it happen.

I hope that by reading this book some of your fears about hospice care will leave. Hospice does not do too many extraordinary things; we just use common sense to do ordinary things extraordinarily well. We celebrate life.

~ Where I Volunteer ~

TO BRIEFLY INTRODUCE the hospice where I have been both a paid marketing employee and a volunteer, *FairHoPe Hospice and Palliative Care, Inc.* is a free-standing, Not-for-Profit (501) 3 (c) hospice that focuses its care in three counties southeast of Columbus, Ohio. In fact, FairHoPe derives its name from those counties: Fairfield, Hocking, and Perry. That is why the "H" and "P" are also capitalized

For most people on hospice service, care is covered by Medicare, the patient's health insurance, or possibly, Medicaid. People on FairHoPe's service uncompensated care is covered through the FairHoPe Hospice Memorial Fund. No one is turned away from FairHoPe Hospice if their live expectancy is six months or less.

People on FairHoPe Hospice and Palliative Care, Inc.'s service are cared for in their homes, wherever they consider home to be. Sometime an alternated plan is needed and that is why FairHoPe opened a twelve-bed inpatient unit, The Pickering House, in February of 2007. Generally, FairHoPe patients are admitted to "The House" for a few days' stay to give respite (a break) for the caregiver. Other reasons for admission include: short-term pain and symptom management, time for care-giving arrangements to be made, or imminent death.

~ A Few Hospice Myths~

THERE ARE MANY myths about hospice care. Most of the myths are a result of not knowing the whole story and, most likely, not *wanting* to know the whole story. Let's face it; talking about the last stage of life isn't always pleasant. But one of the things I've learned in life is to avoid contempt without investigation. I try not to make a judgment about something until I've done a little investigation. So, let's do a little investigating into a few of the myths about hospice care.

Years ago, probably the first thing that I heard about hospice was, "Don't go there, they kill people." You've probably heard, or thought, the same thing. I still hear of people advising someone not to sign on to hospice because they kill people. There have been stories where "They called in hospice and the next day he died." To be truthful that does happen more than it should and for one very simple reason; the person was actively dying when hospice was called. For some, the perception of when to call hospice is just that; when someone is dying. Maybe that thought prevails because if for no other reason, nobody knows what to do when a person is actively dying. It is absolutely a myth that hospice kills people.

The fact is that every hospice gets paid a per diem amount of money from Medicare for each patient on service. "Per diem" means "For each day." Therefore, we get a set amount of money for each day that a patient is on our service. So, our incentive is to have someone on service for a long time in order to get paid for a long time. Sounds like an oxymoron, but we at hospice don't want those on our service to die! In fact, many studies by insurance companies, the government, medical schools, etc. consistently show that people live longer on hospice service than those spending the last stage of their life trying not to die by enduring more treatments. To be honest, since we care for people during the last stage of life, yes, many will die on service, but they usually die later than anybody guessed. Some even sign off because their health improved to the point that they were no longer appropriate for hospice.

Not long ago, the hospice where I volunteer had a man on our service whose story poignantly demonstrates that people live longer on hospice service. He was in his early 40's and his doctor diagnosed him with advanced cancer. The doctor told him that he probably had 5 or so months of life remaining, but gave him some hope by telling him that an experimental treatment might allow him to live up to three months longer. The doctor admitted that there would probably be some side effects from the treatment. Against his doctor's advice, the patient chose hospice compassion and comfort. He lived for 17 months under our care. About twelve months after his admission, he rode with us in the 4th of July parade. His friends along the parade route kept running up to get a quick picture with him. The patient lived many more months than his doctor anticipated and, most importantly, he had fun during those months. When my hospice says, "We celebrate life!" we're not kidding. So, to dispel a very prominent myth about hospice, NO, we don't kill people.

The story about the patient brought up a second myth. That is, hospice only cares for somebody for six months or less. This myth comes from the Medicare requirement that to be eligible for Medicare's Hospice Benefit, a beneficiary must be entitled to Medicare Part A and be certified by a physician to have a life expectancy of *six months* or less if the illness follows its normal course. Many of our patients live more than six months on our service. So what does hospice do when that happens? We keep them on our service, because even the government realizes that it can't predict when someone will die.

The fact is, the status of each patient is reviewed after 90 days, and again their status is reviewed after another 90 days. Those two 90-day periods comprise the six-month period. The Medicare Hospice Benefit consists of two 90-day benefit periods followed by an unlimited number of 60-day benefit periods. Each of the Medicare 60-day benefit periods requires medical recertification.

A fairly recent guideline from the government mandates that a hospice physician or certified nurse practitioner (CNP) must have a face-to-face encounter with each hospice patient to determine their continued eligibility at the end of the 180-day recertification, and prior to each subsequent 60-day recertification. The truth is, the only one who knows how long someone will live is the patient alone.

Well, I hope everyone feels better and sleeps well tonight. We have dispelled two hospice myths. First, we learned that hospice does not kill people because hospice staff is very compassionate and is paid for each day that a patient is on service. Second, we learned that no one is signed off of hospice service if they are still alive after six months. They may stay on service as long as their health seems to be declining.

~ WHEN WAS HOSPICE INVENTED? ~

MY GRANDDAUGHTER RECENTLY asked me, "Papaw, when was hospice invented?"

"Well," I said, "that's not an easy question to answer. The fact is, the hospice movement wasn't invented but evolved slowly over almost a thousand years. Something this good doesn't just happen overnight."

Briefly, Christians established what they called "hospices" during the Middle Ages. These hospices served as places for travelers to rest on pilgrimages to the Middle East. Much later, in 1870, Mother Mary Aikenhed of the Irish Sisters of Charity opened Our Lady's Hospice in Dublin, Ireland, to care only for the dying. This is believed to be one of the first exclusively end-of-life care facilities.

The 1940's were the beginning of the Antibiotic Age. Medical care became more scientific and the inability to cure was viewed as failure. In the 1960's, Dr. Cicely Saunders established St. Christopher's Hospice near London, England, thus initiating the modern hospice movement. The first hospice in America opened in New Haven, Conn, in 1974. Hospice became a Medicare benefit in 1982.

I can bet my bottom dollar that every hospice in the United States has received many praises for the love and compassion given to those families dealing with end-of-life issues. That is because something this good doesn't just happen overnight.

~ Now A Person ~

MOST PEOPLE HAVE been referred to as a "patient" at some point in their adulthood. And most of the people who have signed on to hospice have probably been referred to as a patient for a long time before coming to us. I think that one of the reasons people invariably say, "If only I knew," once they've experienced hospice compassion, is because of the subliminal way we put the "person" back in the patient. We accomplish it by changing the focus from illness, medicine, and treatments to life, relationships, and goals.

Our approach is family-oriented, with the family as the unit of care. During our initial consult, we determine what the ill person wants, not so much what they need. And we then develop our plan of care from that information. It may be as simple as where they want their hospital bed placed if they will be living at home. For example, as a patient-contact volunteer, one of my patients had his bed set up in the Living Room so that he could still be involved in his family's life, plus wave to his neighbors.

Those who don't understand hospice care think that someone on our service is still just a patient. And on government and insurance forms they need to be referred to as a patient, but hospice sees the beauty that is still within. We restore a patient to what they used to be – a living person whose opinion is listened to and acted upon.

Give hospice a call and let us care for the person who is ill.

~ TOTAL COMFORT ~

WE HUMANS ARE three-part beings. We are a combination of body, mind, and spirit, and these parts are all connected. When there is a problem in one of these areas, usually the other two areas also experience problems. The founder of the modern hospice movement, Dame Cicely Saunders, first used the term "Total Pain" to encompass into a whole the individual pain experienced by the body, mind, and spirit. Hospice understands this and approaches the plan of care of the individual on service with all three areas included.

Second to anxiety, I think the root of most misconceptions about hospice is the belief that we are like most other medical organizations, that we are just a continuum of the same thing. We are not. We don't just deal with the disease – we deal with the whole enchilada, so to speak. When a person signs on to a local hospice, each of the three areas of body, mind and spirit is individually addressed.

To illustrate the hospice commitment to the total being concept, three different people are normally involved in evaluating a person when they sign on to hospice. Generally speaking, the intake nurse is concerned with the disease, the social worker is focused on the patient's emotional status, and the chaplain is concerned with their spiritual condition. Depending upon the situation, these visits may be in short order or spread out over several days.

Normally a social worker makes the initial visit in order to determine if the person is, indeed, eligible for our service. Sometimes a nurse will make the first visit if none of our social workers are available. If it is determined that the person is appropriate, the social worker will then discuss any medical directives, learn about the family structure, and the emotional status of those most affected by the situation. Acceptance of the seriousness of the disease is of paramount importance for everyone involved.

Next, one of our nurses will arrive to talk specifically about the patient's history with the ailment and to discuss in general their medical history. The nurse will contact the person's doctor, or doctors, to discuss all the medications the person is taking. Sometimes there may be medicines taken that address the side effects of other medicines being taken. This is a common occurrence. Given the progress of the illness, many of the prescriptions are no longer needed. We may recommend that some medicines be discontinued, but it's up to the person or their family to make the final decision. I need to emphasize that with hospice, especially the one where I volunteer, we let the family make the final decision. Sometimes the best medicine is to teach someone how *not* to need it.

As a side bar, one of the many nice things about our nurses is that they are familiar with many of the area doctors. Often, they have direct access to your doctor and if they don't, they are at least able to make direct contact with your doctor's assistant. This means that they usually get answers quickly.

Continuing with the admission process, after our social worker makes the initial assessment and our nurse has an understanding of the progress of the disease, the medicine being taken, and has consulted with your doctor, the third person to make contact with you is one of our chaplains. It's important to specifically note that at the hospice where I volunteer, chaplains are not calling to witness to anyone or shame anyone who has not gone to church in a while. The chaplain will call simply to inquire about the person's spiritual condition and offer to visit.

Sometimes, when the person has a strong spiritual life, a good church family and a pastor who has been in contact with them, they may decline the visit. No hard feelings. The chaplains find it a comfort to know that the person is spiritually at peace.

But when discussing the fear of all humans, dying, the one question that seems to be on everyone's mind is, "what happens next?" Hospice's chaplains have the time to listen and to talk about what happens next in order to ease the patient's fear of dying. They have the time to help find meaning in the person's life and to use biblical, or other sacred stories, to help the person find their spiritual path. They also have the time to just be there. A patient's daughter once told me that the chaplain just seemed to silently "be" with her mother, as if Jesus was sitting with her.

The end of life is not a medical experience; it is a spiritual experience that can be fraught with fear. As the disease continues, the focus gradually shifts away from the disease until it's no longer in the conversation. The emotional status of the patient slowly lessens until it also is of no importance. Spirituality gains prominence as the end of life approaches until it's the only area of focus. If the family desires, hospice will have a staff member present if the end appears to be imminent, although there is no way to accurately predict when the hour of death has arrived.

The nurse, social worker and chaplain are alert to the fact that each of their areas of expertise may overlap each other. Sometimes the person will tell the nurse that they are afraid of dying because they are worried about their children. Or they may tell the chaplain they feel physical pain, such as headaches, that are a result of emotional tension in the family. The social worker may be told of spiritual pain felt because the physical pain is interpreted as punishment for wrong-doing. Any hospice worker will take the time to listen when these situations arise.

When you contact hospice soon after your diagnosis, you allow yourself time to experience a calmness and serenity rarely experienced in life. That is the total comfort of body, mind, and spirit.

~ A Familiar Word ~

"CAREGIVING" IS A word that I've heard more and more frequently in the last few years. As the Baby Boomers advance through the years, they are now reaching a new threshold in life. Many, like my Mom in the mid-1990's, want to stay home even as they age. And to do so, they will most likely need a caregiver to some degree. In my case, my younger sister was Mom's caregiver. Later, my brother took over the duties. He owned a business and planned to come home when needed. He thought, "Yeah, I can handle this."

Well, he couldn't. With all due respect to his intentions and a deep love for his mother, he just couldn't keep up. Caregiving for Mom was a 24-hour-a-day, no-days-off proposition and he just couldn't do it. I would like to encourage those who are currently immersed in care giving to hang on. If you need help, ask.

In today's society, the term "caregiver" is used extensively to mean someone who is caring for a homebound family member in their home. It is news to no one who is caring for a loved one at home that being a caregiver is very difficult.

The Work and Family Researcher's Network describes caregiving as the act of providing unpaid assistance and support to family members or acquaintances who have physical, psychological, or developmental needs. They state that caring for others generally takes three forms: instrumental, emotional, and informational caring. Instrumental help includes activities such as shopping for someone who is disabled or cleaning for an elderly parent. Caregiving also involves a great deal of emotional support which may include listening, counseling, and companionship. Part of caregiving for others may be informational in nature, such as learning how to alter the living environment of someone in the first stages of dementia.

When taking care of someone at home, the tasks may seem easy at first. As my brother said and I'm sure many have repeated, "Yeah, I can handle this. I don't need any help." Yet, relentlessly the tasks keep coming. They start to come more frequently and they just don't stop. If you are taking care of a spouse, you may change from being a spouse to becoming a resentful servant. Even when not at home, you are worrying. After a while you seem to change from being a human being to a human "doing." If you are a caregiver and you feel stress heighten don't hesitate to ask for help.

There are many facets to caregiving, but one that seems to be universal is compassion fatigue, i.e., what we used to call "burnout." After an extended period of maybe a few months of taking care of someone close, you may get the feeling that you have no life of your own. You are hurrying home after work, then immediately become the caregiver until bedtime. Or, more realistically, you are the caregiver until it's time to go back to work. This can cause resentment or guilt in the caregiver.

How much longer can you keep doing this? Those feelings of resentment and guilt are normal if you are having a down day. If those feelings become the norm, it may be a sign of compassion fatigue. The comedian, Jeff Foxworthy, said that if someone you are caring for asks for their wheelchair and you yell, "Get it yourself!" then maybe you have reached the burnout stage. Remember that God won't give you more today than you can handle. The trick is not to pile on yesterday and tomorrow. That's when it becomes more than you can handle.

Borrowing from Jeff Foxworthy again, there may be a few indicators that you are a caregiver and not someone who is just helping out a little. For example, if you're on a first name basis with the hospital security guard, you may be a caregiver. Or if you use Neosporin as a verb (as in) "I gotta Neosporin this so we can get to church on time," you just may be a caregiver.

I believe it was Josef Stalin who said that one death is a tragedy, but a million deaths is a statistic. I think the same can be said about the countless acts of kindness that constitute caregiving. For a while the acts are so nice, but after a while they aren't noticed. The thought that the person being cared for has no clue about what you gave up to do this can cause resentment to build. The care you give just seems like routine, even expected, to the one who receives it.

Former President Jimmy Carter's wife Rosalyn Carter said that there are four kinds of people in the world: those who have been caregivers, those who are currently caregivers, those who will be caregivers, and those who will need a caregiver. So, I guess that's about everybody. If you're a caregiver, you are not alone.

I've heard it said that a doctor may diagnose an illness and a nurse may try to heal, but it's the caregiver who makes sense of it all. It can however, overwhelm the caregiver. It's important to take care of yourself. If you are at the end of your rope, tie a knot and hang on. Consider asking for help. A little assistance can help put order back in your life.

~ CELEBRATE INDEPENDENCE ~

HAPPY INDEPENDENCE DAY! If you know someone who is on hospice service, you might want to call them and wish them a happy Independence Day because at hospice, every day is Independence Day.

Happy Fourth of July! This holiday was originally known as Independence Day because it was on July 4th, 1776 that the Colonies ratified the Declaration of Independence. "Independence" may be defined as self-rule. This definition applies to either a country or a person. We all know someone who is independent. That is, they don't want others to tell them what they should do.

What we do at hospice is exactly that, we give our patients independence. We don't tell our patients what to do. When someone signs on to hospice compassion, our plan of care starts with the question, "What does the patient want?" After all the months, or years, of having their life ruled by their disease, we throw off the shackles of treatments, restricted diets, side effects and trips to medical facilities. With hospice, when someone accepts our care during the last stage of life (which is six months or less) they are free to eat and drink what they want. They are free to tie up all the loose ends of their past and enjoy a pain-free life. And all of this, including many therapies, at no cost! Isn't that something to celebrate?

After all the problems and heartaches of life, we give our patients their independence by letting them do whatever the heck they want. Now that's something to celebrate!

~ CELEBRATE THE FOURTH ~

DURING THE WEEK before the Fourth, we hear a lot about freedom, liberty and – I hate to say it – sales. Most people don't seem to realize how fragile our freedom is. It's easy to take freedom for granted, when you've never had it taken from you. Additionally, it's also easy to take your health for granted, when you've never had it taken from you. While you're celebrating the birth of our freedom during the Fourth of July, celebrate how lucky you are to be, well, celebrating.

Where I work, we celebrate life. There is no better place to learn about how precious life is than to work where you see it end. There is nowhere better to learn about living life to the fullest than to work where you see it ebbing away. There is nowhere better to celebrate life than to work where everyone there celebrates life.

This holiday is the perfect time to celebrate what is good in your life; good country, good relationships, and good health.

~ CHECK ENGINE LIGHT ~

ONE OF THE misconceptions of hospice care is that some people say we sedate patients to manage their pain. In reality, when physical pain is a symptom of a patient's illness, we let the patient advise us about how much or how little pain medicine they want. But there are more causes of pain than just the physical aspect. There is also emotional pain and spiritual pain. Both of these can manifest as physical pain, such as a tension headache when under stress.

Addressing the possibility of either emotional pain or spiritual pain of a person is one of the many ways that hospice is different from what most people expect. Neither of these types of pain can be properly dealt with by pain medication. Covering up a pain without knowing its cause is like disconnecting the "Check Engine" light on your car. You haven't found the problem but at least the light will quit bothering you. The engine problem may become worse but without a warning light we think everything is okay.

All wounds aren't visible. The crisis of the last stage of life can cause repressed fears and emotional wounds to surface in the guise of physical pain. Once our staff helps a patient cure these invisible wounds, a truly pain-free, serene last stage of life may be enjoyed. Many times, when someone signs on to hospice service soon enough, they live longer than expected. Part of that may be because we don't just unplug the warning light, we take care of the problem.

~ COMMUNICATING DOESN'T JUST MEAN TALKING ~

WHEN I WAS going through my training to be a hospice volunteer, I went through a communication class. Some of the important aspects of communicating that we discussed in that class were to be opened-minded when dealing with people (don't prejudge), to listen (not just wait my turn to talk) and to observe their mannerisms and body language. Seems strange, but talking was not discussed in that class nearly as much as the prejudging, body language and listening.

As an example of non-judgmental, non-verbal communication, a family that I was involved with a few years ago comes to mind. The assignment was that of a man roughly my age. Clearly, he was too young to be in this situation. He had oral cancer and consequently could not talk.

My first visit was on a gloomy, cold, Good Friday evening. I am always apprehensive on my first visit because I don't know what to expect from the patient's personality, the family dynamics, the type and condition of the living quarters, etc. Since I am entering another family's inner sanctum I must be accepting of their way of living. At this stage, I make a conscious effort to be completely open-minded. If I'm not, any of my body language or facial expressions may signal disapproval. Non-verbal communication plays an even larger role in our lives than verbal communication.

The apartment that I entered was where this man had lived for years and it was in this apartment that he chose to complete his life. His room was filled with display cases of swords, daggers, battle-axes and various other types of weapons. Many more similar items were mounted on the walls. Even the patient himself was covered with tattoos of daggers and swords. His hair was combed back in the classic duck-tail style of the 1950's. My first impression was that he must've been a "pretty tough customer" at one time.

As mentioned, he could not speak so I learned in a hurry how he conveyed when he needed his mouth moistened or the TV channel changed. About a half an hour into the visit, his 9-year-old granddaughter arrived, she was a "spittin image" of the girl who played the middle daughter on the 80's sitcom, "Full House." This little girl had the same hairstyle, same voice, and the same looks as the character Stephanie.

After her arrival, she took off her coat, then come over to her Grandpa's bedside. She pulled over a chair, stood up on it, gently raised his head off the pillow, and brushed his hair. She pulled down his blanket and sheet, then brought them back up and tucked them under his chin.

Next, she moistened his lips with a toothette (a small sponge on a stick), wiped his face with a warm wash cloth, changed the TV channel to his favorite show and finally sat down on the chair next to his bed. She tenderly put her hand through the bed railing, placing it on the mattress near his waist.

I thought the patient was asleep because his eyes had been closed and he was passive through all her activity. He slowly moved his hand off his abdomen and onto her hand. As their fingers entwined, I felt a tear form. I was profoundly touched by what I had just witnessed. After a minute, she looked at me and said, "This is how he tells me that he loves me."

Sometimes there are no words to express what is being felt. What I witnessed was love in its purest form. She communicated love to him without saying a word, and he as well. One half hour earlier I had entered a somewhat dingy apartment filled with the acrid smell of stale cigarette smoke. I had entered the room of a gruff-appearing patient. It was a room that was filled with articles of violence. In very short order, in a very quiet way, I had learned about love, tenderness, and communication.

It's easy to get wrapped up in the surface drama of a situation and overlook the silent connection of the eyes or the tender affection of two hands touching. This little girl taught me that to truly communicate all you need is a hand to hold and a heart to understand. I haven't had a hospice family yet who hasn't taught me in some little way that communicating doesn't just mean talking.

~ Don't be Dreary ~

PART OF MY duties as Community Education Coordinator is to present the good news of hospice compassion by means of speaking to groups. I have talked to groups as small as five and larger than 250. I have presented the good news of hospice compassion to cancer support groups, Twigs, car clubs, civic organizations, congregations during Sunday Service, medical groups, senior groups, etc. Sometimes I'm contacted by email, but mostly I am contacted by phone.

Normally, at some point during the initial call to set up the engagement, the caller will casually ask that I not be too dreary when speaking to the group. I'm usually not. In fact, the standard comment that I receive after a speaking engagement is that they never dreamed the presentation could be so uplifting and full of positive stories. Probably the greatest myth of signing on to hospice is that it will be sad and, well, a little dreary.

Hospice respects a family's way of dealing with stress; we don't try to change anything. Most families, however, are surprised to learn that, along with the heartfelt conversations and prayers, the last months of life can be filled with fulfillment, peace, comfort, and even laughter.

I believe that most hospices welcome the opportunity to talk to any group about the goodness of hospice care. Hopefully, they won't be dreary.

~ Enjoy the end of life? ~

PEOPLE DON'T ORDINARILY think of enjoyment when they think of hospice. The truth is, when someone signs on to hospice compassion with more than just a few weeks of life remaining, they can enjoy this stage of life. And this should be the best stage. When you were born, everyone was smiling and you were crying. At the end of life, wouldn't it be nice for you to be the one smiling, and everyone else is crying?

When I was growing up, my family always had dessert after dinner. My Mom was a great cook and baker, although one evening she fixed cow tongue and canned spinach. Leaving the dinner table after eating her apple pie or chocolate cake with fudge icing always gave me a good feeling . . . even if cow tongue and canned spinach were part of the main dinner.

Hospice gives the patient and family time to spend together, something that can't be done in an Intensive Care Unit. I often hear people say that they are going to fight the disease to the bitter end. It's their life and it's their choice. Hospice respects everyone's way of doing things, even if it's to have a bitter end.

One thing we all agree upon is that there *is* an end. Those fortunate enough to sign on to hospice are given the chance to have a nice ending. Yes, with even the chance of having an enjoyable one.

~ Father's Day Gift ~

I F YOU ARE trying to come up with an idea for a different kind of Father's Day gift, consider letting your dad know what he means to you by writing down your thoughts in a letter. Maybe include a photo of him and you. My experience has been that this is a gift a dad will treasure forever. You might simply get a nice photo frame and put inside it a handwritten note telling your dad that he's been a good dad.

For Father's Day several years ago, my four grown children did something different. It was by far the best Father's Day gift I've ever received. It was a photo album in which each of them wrote a one-page letter recalling their favorite childhood memories of spending time with me. They shared memories of regular Saturday morning breakfast at the White Cottage Restaurant on High Street and of hikes up in the woods in the winter to "burn" hotdogs on a campfire. Memories of going to a Cincinnati Red's game every June and of me helping them with math homework.

Although we had gone on vacations to Cape Cod and Virginia Beach, among other places, what they wrote about was the time I spent with them. Each child also picked out their favorite photos of just me with them and placed the photos on the facing page. If I'm allowed one carry-on item when I go to Heaven, I'm taking my Father's Day album.

And dads, remember that to be in your children's memories tomorrow, you have to be in their lives today. Give them your time.

~ Financial Relief ~

THE MEDICAL NEEDS of a patient are what most people think about when battling a serious illness. And, although many won't admit it, "How are we going to pay for all of this?" is a secondary, yet, troublesome concern. Hospice helps the patient and their family not only to work their way through disease issues, but through the financial issues, as well.

The hospice where I volunteer does everything possible to remove all the burdens that a serious illness creates, no matter how small, so that the patient and family can focus exclusively on each other. One of the first things that lets people know problems will be taken care of is that the minute they sign on to hospice compassion, all expenses related to the terminal illness, from that point forward, stop. Oh, what a relief that is!

My hospice handles all the paperwork and all the costs that are associated with the terminal illness. The social worker will contact the patient's insurance company if they have insurance, then Medicare and Medicaid seeking reimbursement for our services. If for any reason the patient doesn't qualify through these avenues, the service is free. Money received from fundraisers such as a 3K Family Memorial Walk in April, a Cookie Walk in December, and various other fundraisers, plus donations, are then used to pay for our services.

Many independent studies by universities and research organizations have shown that people live longer, and yes, are happier, on hospice service. At a time like this, you have enough on your mind. Oh, what a relief hospice is!

~ Ginger Bread Cupcakes with Green Icing ~

ONE OF THE hallmarks of hospice care is that, based on the symptoms of the illness, we allow families to continue living life in as normal a manner as possible. The patient continues to live where they are living and their daily routines and holiday traditions continue. If families have a holiday tradition, we try to work around it so as not to interfere.

St. Patrick's Day is March 17th and for just about everyone who is of Irish decent, this is THE holiday of the year. There are many St. Patrick's Day traditions, even for those who are Irish on this day only. I had a patient who was 100% Irish. Her family had traditions for every holiday. And with St. Patty's Day in March, one tradition that occurred every year was her gingerbread cupcakes with green icing. One of her grown children told me that coming home from school as a first grader, as a freshman in high school, or a freshman in college, there they'd be on two large plates: normal size cupcakes on one plate and the small 1 ½" diameter little ones on the other plate. All of them covered with green icing. Evidently, she was a great baker, but St. Patrick's Day was the only day that she would make gingerbread cupcakes.

Hospice supports the family and allows life to go on as routinely as possible. This woman came on service too late in life to bake any this year. But I know if she had been on hospice service last year, somehow there would have been two plates of gingerbread cupcakes with green icing on the table.

~ Gratitude List ~

AT HOSPICE, WE celebrate life! One definition of "celebrate" is to honor, as in when we celebrate Memorial Day. On that day, we honor the military who have died for our freedom. We show them gratitude.

The difference between *feeling* grateful and *being* grateful is action. One of the volunteers at my hospice, Tracey, helps our families show gratitude to their loved one while they are still alive, rather than telling others at the funeral. To take this idea a bit further, why wait until the end of life? Do it now! Tracey practices what she preaches. To wit: she recently sent me this note:

"Over the weekend, my husband and I traveled to a bordering state to attend my niece's high school graduation party. Months ago, I sent her a letter asking her to write a letter of gratitude to her parents and present it during her party. I enclosed suggestions on how to craft the letter...she embraced the idea."

During the party, my niece asked her father to quiet the crowd. The parents thought she was going to thank the crowd; I knew differently. She kicked off her pumps and stood on a chair. Then, she pulled a hand-written letter from her pocket and proceeded to give a speech honoring her parents and their lessons. My sister's tears flowed and the crowd was stunned."

"What a priceless experience!"

If you can't think of anything that you're thankful that they did, think of what you're thankful that they didn't do. It can be a deeply moving experience for all involved.

~ Have You Turned Around? ~

WHEN I WAS a freshman in high school, a song came out entitled *"Turn Around"* by Dick and DeeDee. Even as a teenager, it made me think of the passage of time. Just recently I heard the song played on an Internet station, KD Radio. I hadn't heard that song for quite a while and it hit me hard for some reason; maybe because it was autumn. That season, autumn, more than any other reminds me of the passage of time. That song, using very few words, conveys the emotion of the passage of time.

Condensing the lyrics written by Malvina Reynolds, the song asks where have you gone, my little one. Turn around you're two, turn around you're four, turn around you are a young girl going out of my door. Turn around you're tiny, turn around you're grown, turn around you're a wife with babes of your own.

I consider myself to be in the autumn of my life. I don't consider that sad. I'm glad I've made it this far. I've turned around when my children were tiny, I've turned around when they were grown and now when I turned around they have babes of their own; grandchildren!

Hospice understands the seasons of life. We are there during your last season of life to offer comfort and serenity in the familiar surroundings of where you live. Our purpose is not to extend life at all cost. Our purpose is to give you, and your family, the time to turn around and reminisce.

~Hospice is Easy ~

HOSPICE IS VERY easy to get along with. One of the reasons I've heard someone say they wouldn't sign on to hospice service is because they're afraid that once they sign on they can't change their mind and sign off of service. Yes, you can, and you may sign off for absolutely no reason whatsoever. We understand the intensity of what is going on and that under such stress it's difficult to sort things out.

The hospice where I volunteer is a not-for-profit organization which means that we are not trying to make a profit. Some hospices are for profit, so yes, they do try to charge for some of their services. We don't have to make a quota or try to make a profit. Our sole purpose is to provide comfort.

If you are on hospice service and hear of an experimental treatment or drug, go ahead and pursue it. But once you initiate any type of curative action for the terminal disease, you are off hospice service. Should the effort prove fruitless, you are welcome to come back on service. There are no penalties or fees for doing so. It's your life and you may choose to do what you want. Hospice does not interfere.

What hospice does is comfort. We comfort physically. We comfort emotionally. And we comfort spiritually. Part of the emotional comfort is to allow you the freedom to do what you think is best and to know that we will always be here to welcome you back should you decide to come back. Hospice is easy to get along with.

~ UNIQUE, JUST LIKE THE OTHERS ~

I OFTEN RECEIVE compliments from people telling me how wonderful hospice care was for their family member. Sometimes, if I don't recognize the name of their loved one, they will tell me something to the effect of, "Oh, they didn't live around here. They lived in Illinois." I'll acknowledge the compliment by telling them I'm happy that they were well cared for. I will then tell them that it isn't the hospice where I volunteer who deserves the compliment but a different hospice. They'll smile and say something to the effect that our nurses, aides, and volunteers were great. They're thinking hospice is hospice and that was just our Illinois office.

One of the many myths, or misconceptions, of hospice is that it's one national medical company. It's not a national company; rather, hospice is a philosophy of care. Each hospice organization follows its own manner of providing hospice centered patient care. As one person quipped, "Your hospice is unique, just like all the other ones." As a comparison of how hospices can be different, think of a fast food hamburger restaurant, or "Quick Service Restaurant," as the industry prefers to be called. Visualize a rectangular building in which you generally enter the parking lot and park in front or to the right of the restaurant.

When you enter most of these fast food hamburger outlets, the ordering counter will be on the left side of the interior and restrooms on the right. The menu board is above and behind the ordering counter. The restaurant also has an outdoor drive up ordering station in back, and one or two windows where you pay and pick up your "drive-thru" order around the left side of the building. I could be describing any one of the three major hamburger fast food brands: Burger King, Wendy's, or McDonalds.

Although fast food hamburger restaurants are regulated by national and local health department guidelines and perform the same basic function, they are vastly different. The same is true of hospice. All hospices perform the same function of caring for people who are terminally ill and all hospices are governed by various government entities. And all hospices receive from Medicare a per diem (a set amount of money per day) for each patient that they have on service. They also may receive money from the patient's insurance. Yet each hospice is vastly different because each approaches the care of patients in their own unique manner.

There are national organizations that a hospice may belong to such as the National Hospice and Palliative Care Organization (NHPCO). This may help create the illusion of one big organization such as the Red Cross. The NHPCO is a non-profit membership organization representing hospice and palliative care programs and professionals throughout the United States. It does not govern any particular hospice. In Ohio, LeadingAge Ohio, formerly Midwest Care Alliance serves the same function for hospices within the State of Ohio. Again, neither of these organizations are governing bodies.

An essential difference in hospice-care and one that essentially splits hospices in America into two groups is the way they are funded. This difference in funding is the basis on how service is provided. The two categories for funding hospice are: for-profit and not-for-profit. That sounds self-explanatory but it's good to understand how they are funded because it can affect what services they provide and how they provide them.

The bottom line is that a for-profit hospice has to make a profit to pay expenses and salaries, and also dividends to shareholders. Not-for-profit hospices need to make a profit, as well, because they, too, have to pay expenses and salaries just like the for-profits do, but they don't have to pay shareholders a dividend like the other group does.

The hospice where I volunteer is a not-for-profit hospice. We are very good stewards of the money we receive. But when a decision is being made about how to address the needs of an ill person or their family, we don't necessarily need to look for a cheaper way of doing things. A not-for-profit has more freedom to do what is necessary to meet the emotional and spiritual needs of a patient with less constraints on the cost. Let's face it; profit isn't a concern for a person nearing the end of life.

Hospice is not so much a medical-oriented operation as it is a relationship and spiritual organization. Emotional and spiritual needs cannot be budgeted into a plan of care. Fundraisers, such as 5K runs, help a not-for-profit provide care for a patient who may need more extensive care than most patients. Fundraisers also allow not-for-profit hospices to care for someone who may not have any means of financial support. Fundraising also helps hospices with various non-budgeted needs. An example of a hospice service not compensated for by insurance or Medicare is expenses for bereavement follow-up care.

Aside from the differences of each hospice organization, one aspect that seems to be consistent in all hospices is that they attract caring, compassionate staff and volunteers. Because of the emotional intensity that is part of working at a hospice, a new employee won't last very long (job wise) at a hospice if they are just looking for a job.

Now that you know that "hospice is hospice" is not an accurate statement, you may want to think about what to do should your doctor gently tell you that there is nothing more that can be done. That "...maybe we should consider calling hospice." Wherever you live remember that hospice, any hospice, is a good thing when facing a potential last stage of life situation. Not all hospices do what I describe in this book, but all hospices do much more than anyone expects.

~ How the Story Ends ~

A RE YOU ONE of those folks who, like me, go to the back of the book to see how the story ends before you begin to read it? I've heard estimates that approximately 40% of people who read short stories and novels start at the back to learn how it ends.

I recently read about a study done at the University of California, San Diego. It concluded that the people who first read the ending of a story enjoyed it more than if they read it from start to finish. The researchers found that knowing how a story ended, even mysteries, didn't hurt the enjoyment but actually improved it for some readers.

The psychologists conducting the study surmised that when reading a book, the reader is subconsciously trying to guess the ending. The tension in not knowing what happens next detracts from the reader's enjoyment. But when the ending is known beforehand the reader sees how all the parts of the plot fit. Although the article about the study did not mention it, I think that is also why we can watch a movie again and again even though we obviously know how it will end. "It's a Wonderful Life" is a good example.

You can be assured that with hospice involved in the last chapter of your Book of Life, you will be provided with a good, pain free, serene ending. Don't be distracted by not knowing how all the pieces of your life fit together. Get out there and celebrate life. Everything's going to be okay.

~ Hospice Chaplains Are Important ~

I was talking with a friend who mentioned to me that being a hospice chaplain would be easy because all you'd have to do is pray with a patient for a few minutes. First, I let him know that for almost everyone involved with the last stage of life, including the ill person, their family, friends, and the medical community, prayer is a very important aspect of the last stage of life. Then I explained that there is much more to being a chaplain at hospice than most people realize.

Well then, what does a hospice chaplain do? My experience has been that the intention of every hospice employee is to comfort the person on service. Probably one of the foremost goals of a chaplain when initially meeting someone on hospice service is to determine their spiritual condition. Coinciding with that is to notice if the person is in any kind of pain: physical, emotional, or spiritual pain.

Our chaplains know that emotional pain may cause spiritual pain and spiritual pain may cause physical pain. As an example, have you ever developed a headache knowing that you have to do something that you are afraid to do? Anticipating giving a presentation, or going to a medical facility to have a procedure done may cause physical symptoms from the emotional distress.

And physical pain may induce spiritual pain. When in physical pain, a person may cry out, "Where are you, Lord? Why are you letting me suffer like this?" Being angry at God at the end of life is quite normal, but this anger may cause the person spiritual pain because they are questioning their spiritual fitness. Our chaplains well understand how the spiritual, physical, and emotional aspects of life blend when we are in a crisis.

Besides our chaplains' primary concerns for the patient's spiritual comfort, they are also interested in their religious beliefs.

There is a difference between spirituality and religion. I've heard the difference described this way – religion is for people who don't want to go to hell and spirituality is for people who have been there. And if you've ever suffered physically or emotionally for an extended amount of time, you understand that definition.

When initially meeting a new person on service, the chaplain will first evaluate their spiritual situation and beliefs. Are they Christian? Did they attend church before the illness worsened? If so, what denomination? This understanding of the spiritual condition is merged with their religious beliefs and practices as a way to ensure they will have spiritual comfort. The hospice where I volunteer uses a non-denominational approach. Our sole purpose is to comfort; we don't convert. All the chaplain wants to do is learn what brings the patient spiritual comfort and respond accordingly.

If they have a church family, the chaplain will contact their pastor. If the illness has kept them from church for a lengthy period of time, we will contact their pastor or if appropriate, contact a different pastor of the patient's denomination. I'm sure that with most hospices, chaplains are familiar with pastors of various denominations who have made themselves available when such a situation arises.

Being a chaplain for hospice doesn't always have to be so serious. One of our chaplains asked a patient, who didn't attend church and initially declined a visit, what she wanted that would comfort her. She replied, "A lottery ticket." Had her health not declined so quickly the chaplain probably would have bought one for her. The chaplain added that the patient was also an avid bingo player so things might have gotten interesting.

There is no rehearsal to prepare a family for what happens when a member is at the end of life. For this reason, the presence of the chaplain can be reassuring. The family is in a crisis and sometimes may be unsure about what to say or do. A chaplain can softly offer guidance. This guidance may include helping the family of a patient make the final good-bye possible.

I remember when my mother was actively dying, we didn't realize it was happening at the time. My wife, a nursing home nurse, recognized what was going on and advised me and my siblings that this was it and that we should tell Mom good-bye. Starting with my oldest brother each of us took as much time as needed in order to say the final goodbye to Mom. Everything happened so suddenly; there was no time to think about it. I took ten minutes and somewhat reminisced about my memories of her and how she was always there when needed. And I had to admit to her that, yes, during my teen years she was usually right. I think that she briefly, faintly smiled at that last comment.

One of our chaplains told me of a family that she was helping. The family gathered around their mom's bedside and each said what they needed to say. The mom, who was at the end of life, lay motionless in her bed while each one said their good-byes. When her son had finished, the woman surprised everyone by sitting up and telling her son, "I love you bunches." Later that evening, through tears, the son told our chaplain, "When I was young, after Mom tucked me in bed at night, she always said, 'I love you bunches.'" Hearing this confirmed with the chaplain how important it was for this family to say good-bye to their mom.

Some people on hospice service don't want a chaplain to visit. That is their choice. A chaplain visit is not required, it is just required to be offered. One patient declined the chaplain visit because she'd heard enough of "that sick and dying kind of talk." When the chaplain suggested that they could just tell each other bad jokes, the patient accepted the visit.

A hospice chaplain does more than anyone would imagine. Personally, I think that the chaplains where I volunteer don't consider what they do a job as much as it is a love for Jesus. They are there to quietly, gently help the people and their families on hospice service. By being available, day and night, to assist and guide those in the crisis of their life, they are the essence of hospice.

~ Let's Live a Little ~

HEY, YOU WANT to have a good time? Ever think about calling hospice? No one ordinarily thinks of enjoyment when they think of hospice. Truthfully, depending on the terminal disease, when someone signs on to hospice compassion, it *is* possible to have a good time. We focus on eliminating the physical, emotional, and spiritual pain. When that is accomplished most patients (and their families) experience a sense of calm and, yes, are even given the opportunity to enjoy life.

Most hospices do not sponsor any type of Bucket List endeavor or special wish type of event, but at the same time, most hospices won't restrict their patients if they'd like to do something "they've always wanted to do." Our employees and volunteers on their own initiative have occasionally helped a patient, and their family, accomplish a desired goal. For example, staff and volunteers have assisted patients in going to the World War II Memorial, visit family in Mexico, and go to an oceanfront resort in Florida. In every parade that my hospice is entered, there is usually a patient riding on our entry.

I often hear people say that they are going to fight it to the bitter end. It's their life and their choice. But one thing we all agree upon is that there is an end. Some just prefer to have a bitter one. After you've exhausted all curative options, consider hospice while there are still months of life remaining. We'll give you the chance to possibly get out and live a little.

~ Should We Call? ~

FROM WHAT I'VE heard, when someone suggests "maybe we should call hospice," the first response most likely is, "Oh no you don't! We're going to fight this to the end." The folks who are a part of hospice understand that calling hospice is usually not the family's first choice. On the other end, with most of the families that I have talked to, someone in the family will lament, "I wish we had called hospice sooner."

Anyone who has been a caregiver of someone seriously ill knows that eventually you get to the point where enough is enough. The illness keeps progressing and nothing is working anymore. The doctor will say, or at least hint, that there is nothing more that can be done.

In this situation, there are only two choices: A) fight it to the bitter end, in which the ill person will have a bitter end, or B) take an unbearably difficult step and call hospice. One of the nice things about choice "B" with most hospices is that if you change your mind later you may sign off with no charge. At least while under hospice's loving care you and your family are able to have a reprieve from all of the tension, physical pain, inconvenience and financial burden of fighting it to the bitter end.

So, here we are. The most difficult step in being on hospice service is to make that first contact with us. To call hospice seems like you are just giving up, but you aren't giving up. You are now beginning to deal not only with the illness; you are beginning to deal with the emotional and spiritual effects of the illness.

A very serious illness not only affects the patient, but has an effect on family and everyone the ill person knows. Hospice is available to comfort all those touched by the illness, even the family pet. Both the family dog and the cat are often distressed by what is going on. I'm not sure if the fish are concerned, though.

When the initial call is made to most hospices you'll notice that an actual person answers the phone – 24 hours a day. Your call is so important to my hospice that we actually answer the phone. And it's okay to cry. Then we ask where you would want to meet to further discuss your situation. Notice that you don't come to our office; we meet in the location of your choosing. That is the first indication that we are nothing like any organization that you've experienced before. And if you can't meet with us during normal daytime hours, we will meet with you in the evening, or on a Saturday or Sunday. If you call near a holiday, we will meet you before, during, or after the holiday. This includes Christmas. Hospice understands that in the last stage of life, the calendar and the clock become less relevant.

Most hospices will meet with you to talk about your situation in your home, where you work, in a restaurant, a hospital or in a park. It's completely up to you. At the hospice where I volunteer, one of our social workers met with the daughter of a prospective patient where she bartended. The daughter couldn't afford to take time off so our social worker met with her during her break at the tavern. There is no pressure to accept. By law, the decision to accept hospice belongs to the patient, or their legal medical care representative.

If you agree to try hospice, it's comforting to know that you may discontinue service at any time. Sometimes people want to try a new treatment. As a patient care volunteer, I went to a regularly scheduled visit of a patient one afternoon. The neighbor met me at the curb and told me the patient and spouse left the previous day to go to a research hospital for an experimental treatment. They were simply removed from our service. They were welcomed back several weeks later. There is no charge to sign off and no charge to sign back on. Medicare and most private insurance companies will allow additional coverage for this purpose.

Once you've agreed to try hospice service one of the first things we will do is contact your physician to make sure he or she agrees that hospice care is appropriate for you at this time. Medicare requires that two physicians need to agree that the patient is appropriate for hospice care. Alternately, it only takes one Hospice Certified Physician to confirm that a patient is, or isn't, appropriate for hospice care.

As the process continues, you will be asked to sign consent and insurance forms. These are similar to the forms patients sign when they enter a hospital. The "Hospice Election Form" states the patient understands that the care is palliative and not curative. "Palliative" in a nutshell means care without curing.

The paperwork will outline all the services available. The form Medicare patients sign also tells how electing the Medicare Hospice Benefit affects other Medicare coverage for a terminal illness. The hospice social worker often assists the family with these forms.

Following the paperwork, the Case Manager, a Registered Nurse who will be the family's primary medical contact, will visit and assess your medical needs. She (or he) will then call your doctor requesting your medical records. During the admission process the third person who visits, after the social worker and nurse, is the chaplain. The chaplain will assess your spiritual situation and call your clergy if you'd like. Some people will decline the chaplain's visit while some want the chaplain to visit on a regular basis.

If you live in a house, the hospice social worker and nurse will evaluate your physical care needs, make suggestions about what durable medical equipment (DME) you'll need, and help you to make arrangements in obtaining any of the necessary equipment.

The process for signing on is easy, but can be emotionally draining. Many have told me that they experienced a profound sense of relief and peace when it was completed.

So, to answer the question of when should you call hospice, "now" is the best answer, before you are in a crisis. Just call us and maybe stop by the office. Bring whoever you want with you, and someone from that hospice can discuss what they do.

I understand this isn't the most pleasant situation to talk about, but at least now you know a little about the process of signing on to service. Each hospice is a little different, but all hospices are dedicated to your comfort. Everything is going to be okay.

~ Acceptance ~

I HAVE FOUND that acceptance is the answer to all my problems. Granted, there have been times the answer might not be the one I was hoping for. But when I surrender to a situation or set of circumstances that I cannot change, life gets easier. Sounds pretty simple, doesn't it?

I remember many years ago, I worked for a robotics company. This was in the early 1980's and the technology pundits were predicting that robots were going to take over the manufacturing world. People were saying that maybe the Jetsons were right.

I was excited to work at a company making robots that were to be used in the manufacture of automobiles. We were even featured in a cable TV news show about robots in our future. Working in a new company in an emerging field was exciting. I knew that my future was secure. After a year, I'd advanced from working in the parts room to being a buyer. Next stop was purchasing agent.

On a cold Friday morning in February, I decided to walk back to the shop floor and check on incoming shipments. Everyone was crying. I thought that one of our employees had died. They said that most of them had just been fired. I soon learned that the investors who were financing the company were not getting a quick enough return on their investment. The decision was made to start over and at least 75% of the employees were let go. Only a few were to stay on in order to get the company back in shape. I felt bad for everyone.

As I was talking to them I was paged over the loud speaker to report to the Personnel Office. I figured that I was being demoted from buyer back to the parts room. When I walked into the office I was handed a pink sheet of paper that said I had 15 minutes to clean out my desk and leave the building. I was stunned, then angry. The worst part was an underling was waiting to escort me to the door.

That afternoon, when I was at home on what should have been a busy Friday at work, I was in shock. I was numb. Pleading for my job was of no use. The decision was made by the investors, not my boss. I had to accept that fact and begin the very unpleasant tasks of filing for unemployment benefits and looking for a new job.

I learned a lot about acceptance that day. Honestly, I had no other choice. The first thing I learned was to accept the present circumstances as they were. Someone once described it as I had to stop barking and start biting. This was a situation where I had no control; I couldn't run from it or fight it. Acceptance was my only choice.

Accepting a new reality, even if it's less good than the one that existed before, such as what happened to me, allows you to live life to the fullest. To use an old cliché, sometimes life forces you to make the best of a bad situation.

That reminds me of the joke in which a woman tells the psychiatrist that her husband thinks he is a chicken. The psychiatrist tells her to bring him in and he'll cure the man. Later the woman calls the psychiatrist saying that she's changed her mind. She'd rather keep her husband the way he is, saying, "Lord knows we can use the eggs."

If you have been given bad news and are in an unpleasant predicament, you can fight it. You can scream about what you've lost, or you can accept it and try to put together something that is good. Quite often after someone has been on hospice service, a family member will tell me, "If only we knew. If only we knew how hospice could have helped us, we would have called sooner."

The terminally ill patient may be accepting of their situation. Maybe they feel that they have lived a full life and have fulfilled their purpose. Maybe they are so sick and tired of being sick and tired that they just want it to end. Or maybe they can accept the terminal diagnosis intellectually but not emotionally.

Often it seems that it's the family who is not accepting of the situation. One or more of the family members just don't want to lose their loved one. That is very normal. But the hard part comes when someone deep down inside the family, like the patient, knows that there is no hope of recovery, yet they just can't bear to lose them. That is where acceptance comes in. At some point, it's a matter of letting go and letting God. The hard part is knowing when.

When a serious illness develops and you are told that curing it isn't possible, you have a choice to fight on anyway or to surrender to it. Hospice does not discourage anyone from pursuing treatment. I know that never surrendering is a choice and many find it a noble one. That is a very personal choice. However, I've found that if something cannot be changed, acceptance makes life easier.

Someone told me that surrendering is like riding the bus facing the direction it's going. Acceptance, thus surrendering, to something that cannot be changed is always an option whether you're a fighter or not. What some consider defeat may actually open the door to peace and serenity. Life can again be good.

Personally, almost a year after my layoff, my life did become good again and I did resume my career. But during that layoff period, in order to help financially, I made little kitchen sets consisting of a child-sized stove, sink and refrigerator. I sold them through the holidays. Almost a decade after that I was pulled over by a city policeman. He was an acquaintance of mine but he had a reputation for giving even his mom a ticket. He told me that he was going to have my car impounded because my license plate was expired.

Then suddenly he said, "Years ago my wife divorced me and gave me custody of our daughter. The only thing my daughter wanted to bring to my house was that kitchen set we bought from you when she was little. That set helped my daughter get through a very rough period for her. I thank you." He then advised me to leave the car where it was and hurry to the License Bureau or else he was going to have my car towed by evening.

I didn't tell you that before he pulled me over I was leaving a yard sale, went only about two houses and turned the corner when he got me. Besides the expired plate, he also cited me for not using my turn signal, not having my seat belt fastened, my driver's license had also expired and he thought that I seemed to be " ...in a little bit of a hurry." I never in a million years would have guessed that one of the many little kitchen sets that I made would have touched a seemingly callous individual to the degree that 10 years later he would extend a kindness to me; a kindness that he probably wouldn't have extended to his own mother.

Should you be in a crisis, know that you will get through it. Things may work out in a way that you never would have dreamed. If you are experiencing a medical crisis, hospice is always available to answer questions. Our primary purpose is to offer comfort, whether it be physical, spiritual, or emotional comfort.

The Serenity Prayer sums up how to handle so many tough situations in life. The short version seems most appropriate here: *God, grant me the serenity to accept the things I cannot change, the courage to change the things I can and the wisdom to know the difference.*

~ Definitely Not a Mistake ~

THERE MAY BE some lively deliberations when a family is discussing the care plans for a seriously ill family member. Emotionally charged statements such as, "Fight it to the bitter end," and, "Never give up," are voiced. "The doctor said the disease can't be cured, it's no use," may also softly be mentioned. One of our social workers has told me that on several occasions she's heard a family member say, "Why would you call hospice? That's a mistake. We won't give up."

For over the twenty years that I've been a patient-contact volunteer with a local hospice, I think that at every funeral I've attended, "If only we knew," is the one phrase consistently heard when discussing the care that hospice gave. Families are quickly filled with gratitude when they experience the all-inclusive love and compassion they receive from hospice staff and volunteers.

Should you be hesitating in calling hospice because of a very serious illness, call us anyway. We will only outline the services we offer. We won't try to force you into a decision. And should you decide to accept your local hospice's compassion, you may cancel at any time and for no other reason than just because you want to. With mine and probably all other hospices, there is no charge to sign on and there is no charge to sign off.

I fully understand that when a loved one is extremely ill, calling hospice is a very difficult decision. Please know that those who have called say that it was definitely not a mistake.

~ THE CAVALRY IS HERE ~

I HAVE HAD patient family members tell me that once they called hospice and signed on for our assistance, they got the feeling that the cavalry had arrived. Meaning that they felt protected and assured when hospice staff and volunteers became involved in the care and comfort of their family member. Why is that? I think one of the reasons is that hospice puts order into what was chaos.

Hospice enters a family's life with everything needed to support a family who has a terminally ill member. We have doctors on staff who will work with your family doctor, or on behalf of your family doctor, to give the best possible comfort. All hospices have chaplains available to assist people who don't have a church family. Or the chaplains may assist the patient's pastor, or they may not be involved at all. We have social workers who assist with medical directives, i.e.; Do Not Resuscitate (DNR) orders, Power of Attorney, etc.

Hospice nurses visit the patient on a regular basis and hospice home health aides may assist with care of the patient. We can order prescriptions and medical supplies and have them delivered in very short order. Hospice offers volunteers who, by their presence, allow caregivers to leave the home and be assured that their loved one is in good hands.

Hospice offers compassion to a family who most likely has been experiencing confusion, tension, and a high dose of fear of the unknown due to a life-threatening illness. Your local hospice has the expertise to put order into what was chaos and to let you get the feeling that the cavalry is here.

~ BACK IN CONTROL ~

ONE OF THE misconceptions, or myths, of hospice is that it's a place; some sort of medical building. The notion is that if you sign on to hospice service you will have to go somewhere. With many hospices, you don't go anywhere. In fact, you stay where you live, whether it's your home, a family member's home, a friend's home, a nursing home, or an assisted living facility.

However, not to muddy the waters, there are some hospices in America that do operate care facilities for their patients. When the famous Washington Post columnist, Art Buchwald, admitted himself into a Washington D.C. area hospice, he moved into their facility. That particular hospice didn't visit their patients in their home like the hospice where I volunteer does. Our hospice facility is, at its core, a short-term respite facility.

And when we care for people who live in their house, we understand that it's their house and not ours. Therefore, they may have their bed set up wherever they want. As a FairHoPe volunteer, several of my patients preferred to sleep in their living room recliners because they were more comfortable. It's their home, after all.

In your home, the feeling of who is in control is brought back to you. In a hospital, or in any type of institution, you are not in control. In your home, you are in control and can stay in any room you prefer. During this stage of your life, being in control is one of the most important aspects of life.

~ The Old Mattress ~

SEVERAL YEARS AGO, a woman reluctantly signed on to the hospice where I am a volunteer. The main reason that she was hesitant to accept hospice care is that she didn't want to leave her home. She felt that she had given up enough as her illness and her age forced things from her hand. She just couldn't move from the home where she had raised her family. Once she understood that under hospice care she would be allowed to remain in her home, she agreed to accept our service. Now the only question remaining in her plan of care was where she wanted the hospital bed placed in her home.

"Hospital bed!? Nope, no hospital bed!" she emphatically said. She couldn't sleep in them. In no uncertain terms, she told us that she would sleep in her own bed, thank you very much. Understand that not all patients living at home under hospice care require a hospital bed, but for her safety a hospital bed was a necessity. Her hospice nurse determined that the problem was she didn't want to give up her old down-filled mattress. She'd slept on this mattress her entire life and she wasn't going to change now. After some discussion, a compromise was reached; the hospital bed would have to be brought in but then they would place her old down-filled mattress on top of the hospital bed's mattress. She was happy.

The last stage of life is uncharted territory so keeping everything familiar is very comforting. When discussing a new person's plan of care, the first question with hospice is, "What does the patient want?" Sometimes it's as simple as a lumpy old down-filled mattress.

~ The Medicine was Taken Away ~

ONE OF THE myths, or misconceptions, about hospice compassion is that once you sign on to our service, you will be taken off all your medications. So many times, when someone signs on to our hospice service they have been taking a primary medication that offered hope of a cure, or at least stabilization of symptoms. When it became frighteningly obvious that it was no longer effective, the ill person might then decide to sign on to hospice. The hospice medical staff will then review the list of medications that the patient has been taking. Invariably the patient will be taking a primary medication and also several medications that were addressing the side effects of the primary medication.

Rest assured that there is no carte blanche policy to remove a patient's medications. Everything hospice does is on a patient-by-patient basis. I think that the reason people believe the myth is because if you hear of someone signing on to hospice service, you may also hear, "...then they took the medicine away."

The fact is, as mentioned previously, the patient and their family are included in any medicine-focused decisions. The hospice medical staff will review all medications that the patient is currently taking and then discuss with the patient (if competent) and family what medicines we feel aren't necessary, and why. Only then will it be decided what medications, if any, should be discontinued. Sometimes the regimen is not changed.

Remember, with most hospices when someone signs on to service, you won't hear, "Of course, they took the medicine away," unless the patient or family helped make the decision to do so.

~ This Just Can't be Happening ~

A S MY MOM'S health began to change for the worse, my fears began to increase. "What if….?" I'd stop abruptly before thinking what I knew deep down was inevitable. "This just can't be happening, not Mom." She had told all of us kids that she would never go to a nursing home. But with increasing frequency, the police would bring Mom back to my brother's home where she was now staying. She had developed a tendency to wander off in the middle of the night. We had no other choice but to place her in a nursing home.

When I drove home after every visit, tears would form. I could tell that Mom was declining and that there was no cure for what afflicted her. What caused those tears was anticipatory grief. I knew my mom was dying and I was grieving as if she had already died. This grief quietly began as soon as I became aware that death was a likelihood.

I was not familiar with hospice when this was happening, but I have since learned that hospice can comfort and support someone when they, too, are thinking that this just can't be happening. And there are other organizations that can help with anticipatory grief; the American Cancer Society and the Alzheimer's Association are two.

If someone close to you is seriously ill, life can be such a confusing, upsetting time. If you are told, "There is nothing more that can be done," remember that hospice has something more it can do. Offering comfort during anticipatory grief is one of them.

~ Volunteers ~

FIVE PERCENT OF the man-hours of care provided by every hospice are mandated by Medicare to be provided by volunteers. This is, to my knowledge, the only area of the health care field that mandates volunteers to be a part of the mix. You may think that the purpose of the mandate is to be a cost-saving measure for a not-for-profit organization. That is not the case. The fact is, hospice developed through the work of volunteers. Initially hospice was largely a volunteer movement. It evolved as a response to the attitude that there was nothing more that could be done when someone was diagnosed with a terminal illness.

Because they are from the general public, volunteers bring in fresh ideas and enthusiasm to every area where they serve. Volunteers act as a liaison between the community and hospice. They bring the community to hospice and in return, bring hospice to the community. There couldn't be a better arrangement.

Occasionally, someone will mention to me that they like the idea of being a hospice volunteer, but don't like the idea of death. That is okay because there are many areas of volunteering that don't involve contact with the patient. Each hospice has its own volunteer program and all programs have areas of need that do not include contact with the patients or families.

Sometimes, volunteer assignments may be tailored to suit individual interests or abilities, possibly developing into a full-fledged volunteer program. The hospice where I volunteer has a children's grief program developed by a volunteer who worked in the education system.

I've been told that volunteering in hospice is a calling. Well, do you feel called?

~ WE HAVE TIME ~

TIME IS MOST precious and savored in the last stage of life, so we don't spend time on things that a person with an apparently longer life expectancy would. When a patient "fights this disease to the bitter end" (which is their right), even though everyone agreed that it couldn't be cured, they are probably using time fighting the disease that could be better enjoyed at home. They are spending time driving to a treatment, or driving to a specialists' office for more tests to confirm what is already known. Maybe another scan to prove that, yes, the tumor is still growing, "Just as we thought."

Numerous independent studies over the last 25 years have shown that people live longer in hospice care. Why? Because we put the person back in the patient and allow them to decide their own comfort level while we actively help them to **enjoy** life.

People who work in hospice understand that there are many tough decisions to make when facing a life-limiting situation. It can be overwhelming and it may seem that time is running out. If you ever get to the point of considering hospice, we'll give you all the time you need if you want to talk things over.

~ We Help Remove Fear ~

I WAS TALKING to my neighbor and he mentioned that he doesn't particularly like talking about the end of life. I can understand that because all of us have a natural fear of dying. But if you are lucky enough to learn that because of an illness, you are entering the last stage of life, each day will become more intense, more precious. If the illness allows, why not enjoy your life? Suffering the after-effects of one more treatments that may actually not extend life is not enjoying life.

Much of what hospice care provides does not involve medicine. Hospice comforts the person's physical pain, emotional pain, and spiritual pain. All three areas are equally important at the end of life. When someone accepts hospice, the patient's care team concentrates on removing each area of pain, at which point life becomes a precious gift to both the patient and their family.

Besides "normal" care, most hospices make available many therapies to enhance one's life. Therapies might include massage therapy, pet therapy, and music therapy. I was recently at a funeral service in which Erin, one of our Music Therapists, talked to those in attendance. She mentioned how the deceased person had taught her his favorite old hymn, one of the few hymns she was not familiar with. She related how she now sings this hymn to other patients, thus carrying on the man's legacy.

Hospice can help remove fears by opening people's eyes to the preciousness of life and help them to live it.

~ It's Life Expectancy, Not Disease ~

"HOSPICE, WE'RE NOT just for cancer anymore!" That sounds like a catchy new advertising slogan, doesn't it? The fact is hospice care never was just for cancer patients. Hospice is, and always was, for end of life care regardless of the disease or illness.

When the hospice movement developed in the late 1960's, cancer lent itself to hospice care. During that era, a cancer diagnosis was like receiving a one-way ticket because the assumption was that there would be no return trip to health. The different types of cancer each followed their own somewhat predictable path, so it was possible to give an estimated life expectancy.

Well then, who qualifies for hospice care? The one sentence that admits someone to hospice care is uncomplicated: A person is eligible for hospice when the primary physician feels that if the disease, or illness, follows its natural course there is six months, or less, of life remaining. Notice that no medical condition is mentioned by name. The *only* criteria is that the physician feels there is six months, or less, of life remaining. And six months is just an educated guess. Over the years, the hospice where I volunteer has had a few patients on service over a year because their health continued to decline and they remained hospice appropriate.

As of this writing, recent statistics have shown that the average hospice caseload has hovered around 50% cancer patients with the balance being a variety of heart, lung, and kidney ailments. Alzheimer's disease and dementia also qualify as being hospice appropriate and those two are becoming more prevalent in hospice.

When facing a life-limiting illness, consider hospice. We're not just for cancer anymore.

~ You Can't Call Too Soon ~

B Y FAR, THE number one phrase that I hear when talking to someone about their experience with hospice is, "If only I knew." Once a person has experienced how hospice calms what can be the greatest emotional crisis in a family's history, they always regret that they didn't call sooner.

I was talking to a woman whose dad was on our service. She said the hardest part of calling hospice was picking up that "100 lb. phone." She described a scenario that I've heard from others when trying to avoid the inevitable phone call to hospice. Everyone who is charged with making that difficult phone call goes through the same thought process of "Should I or shouldn't I?"

The woman told me of the internal argument she had with herself, "No, better not call…got to… can't." She thought it might be better to wait until tomorrow so that way she'd have more facts. Besides, what was the hurry? She said one of her fears was, "What if I called hospice, then found out in a few days that I didn't need to?"

I inquired, "If I understand you correctly, you meant that you were afraid of calling hospice too soon?" She replied that maybe she was. In reality, fear of calling too soon is a very common hesitation for not calling hospice.

I told her that you can't call hospice too soon because no one can be admitted to hospice service unless they meet Medicare guidelines. And, no matter when you sign on to hospice, you can revoke at any time and for no reason whatsoever. There is no charge to sign on and no charge to sign off. Truthfully, there is no risk in calling too early.

One of the good reasons to sign on earlier rather than later is that when someone signs on soon enough there is a chance that they will be discharged from service because their health improved. Our holistic approach to comforting body, mind and spirit creates a serene, calming effect on the person. Since the family is deeply affected by the situation, they receive attention from us, as well. The tranquility hospice brings can work wonders.

When in the throes of fighting a serious illness, there is always the hope that one more procedure will turn things around. The question that has to be honestly answered is, can we or can't we cure the disease? If not, consider calling hospice to see what is offered.

Doctors usually know when the last stage of life has been entered. It's accepting the situation on the emotional side that holds everything up. Your heart may need some time to accept what you may already know deep down.

Something else to think about is that many not-for-profit hospices do not collect for their services; rather, financing is obtained through reimbursement from Medicare, private insurance, fundraisers, and donations. Asking what it will cost when calling hospice is generally a question that rarely comes up during such an emotionally charged phone call. But if you check around before a crisis hits, you may be surprised. The hospice where I volunteer, and others like it, do not charge. When you accept help from such a hospice, you will not spend anything on the terminal illness. Your sole focus will be on the family member who is ill.

In hospices such as mine, we make all the phone calls, contact the doctor and any specialists regarding your hospice decision, and help you with any advanced directives forms. We also order, and set up any durable medical equipment you may need for your home. We will discuss with you all the medicines being taken and will order, deliver, and pay for all prescriptions related to the terminal illness. We will pretty much take care of all the myriad of things that come up when dealing with this type of situation.

The right time to call hospice might be hard to determine. It is good to know, however, that you can't call too soon. Today might be a good day, especially if life is calm. I know that sounds like you're looking for trouble by calling so early in the process, but now is the time to learn. As I've mentioned, when talking to family members, invariably the biggest regret is that they didn't call sooner. My prayer is that you never have to say, "If only I knew."

~ Palliative Care ~

MANY HOSPICES HAVE "....and Palliative Care" at the end of their name. Have you ever wondered about the last word – Palliative? Just what is "Palliative Care?"

Palliative (pronounced Pal-ee-uh-tiv) is basically defined as care without curing. Meaning the patient is cared for but the disease is not the focus. The focus of palliative care is to deal with the side effects of the treatments being administered while pursuing curative measures for a serious illness. In many situations, palliative care gives the patient a second chance to get back to enjoying life even in the face of a chronic illness.

Yes, the patient will receive relief from symptoms such as pain, shortness of breath and fatigue. But when I talk to someone who has had experience with palliative care, what I hear consistently is that on palliative care, the patient now has someone to talk to. One of our palliative nurses has told me that many times the underlying side effect is something as basic to human nature as the need for emotional support.

As far as the nuts and bolts of palliative care it's for someone with a chronic, meaning incurable, disease. Care can be provided at any stage of the illness and curative treatment is continued right along with palliative care. Generally, someone is appropriate for this type of care when their life expectancy is estimated to be around two years.

It may be difficult to decide if you need palliative care. It may be right for you if you suffer from pain or other symptoms due to treatment of a serious illness. There are quite a few diseases that may be chronic. These include: Alzheimer's, Cardiac disease, ALS, cancer, and HIV/AIDS. There are other diseases as well, so it is always advisable to discuss your situation with your doctor.

How does palliative care work? Just fine is the short answer. The palliative care team works with your own doctor to provide supplemental support, in essence, to be the liaison between the doctor and the person who is ill.

Our palliative nurse has told me that she has received thank you notes and phone calls from physicians thanking her for her monthly palliative report about their patients. The reason being that palliative care, like hospice care, focuses on the patient; who they are, where they live, what they are thinking. This insight gives the physician an understanding of the patient that could not have been obtained any other way. The Palliative nurse has the time to spend with the patient to get to know them. By sharing this knowledge through monthly reports, the doctor is able to more deeply understand the emotional status of the patient.

The palliative team provides expert symptom management, extra time for communication and help navigating the health system. In many ways, the palliative team acts as a consultant for you. And, as mentioned above, the monthly report helps the doctor understand more deeply the emotional status of the patient.

In order to receive palliative care, you do not have to go to a clinic or a palliative specialist's office. Palliative care is provided where you live. It may also be provided in the hospital. That aspect of care is such an asset to the patient because so many people appropriate for palliative care are bedbound.

Most insurance plans will reimburse physicians and nurse practitioners for palliative care consults and visits. The hospice where I volunteer, however, offers palliative care as a community support to enhance the patient's quality of life. Because it is a community service, we absorb all our costs and do not charge the patient for the care provided.

Not only does the patient receive relief from pain and fatigue, they can also expect relief from symptoms such as shortness of breath, fatigue, constipation, nausea, loss of appetite and difficulty sleeping. Palliative care helps you carry on with your daily life. It improves your ability to go through medical treatments. It helps you better understand your condition and your choices for medical care. Most importantly, it supports the patient emotionally and spiritually at a time when those two areas are the most important facets of someone' life.

In short, you can expect the best possible quality of life. In addition to expert symptom treatment, palliative care focuses on clear communication, advanced planning, and coordination of care.

As mentioned before, palliative care is usually administered by a team of experts, and it truly is a team. On the patient's team are a palliative care certified doctor, nurse, and social worker. A chaplain, massage therapist, pharmacist, nutritionist, pet therapist and music therapist may also part of the team. While under palliative care, hospice will collaborate with skilled nursing services, home health agencies and physical therapists. You may also go to the hospital for aggressive treatment.

To receive palliative care, it's just a matter of asking your physician to make a referral to the hospice you prefer. Tell your doctor, nurse, family, and caregivers that you want palliative care. You can also call the hospice directly and they can contact your doctor for you.

Life always offers you a second chance. If you know of someone who has been suffering, or maybe it's you, think of palliative care. It can give you a second chance at enjoying life. Palliative care may be just what the doctor ordered.

~ F.A.S.T. Scale ~

I LOVE THE local county fair. The hospice where I volunteer sets up a display in the Arts & Crafts Hall every year at this fair. I've always thought how nice it would be if each of my hospice's staff could spend a few hours at our booth, as I have. It is a pleasant experience to talk to everyone as they stop by.

While at our booth, I get to hear the many compliments about our service and I have a chance to answer questions about parts of our service that aren't understood. By doing so I, hopefully, dispel some of the misconceptions and myths some have about what hospice "really does" when you call them. Through my writing, my goal is to address as many of the rumors and myths as I can. I also try to inform you, the reader, about the many ways hospice can be of service that you may not have been aware of.

While talking to a woman who stopped by the booth, the subject of my newspaper column came up. I told her that the deadline for the next column was only a day away and I couldn't think of a topic to write about. She suggested that I write about what I hear from others at the fair. Maybe write about their experience with hospice or maybe write about a few of the myths that they may bring up. She hit the nail on the head because several of my columns have been based upon a comment or a story from visitors to our booth at the county fair.

One of the subjects that has come up more often in recent years is Alzheimer's disease. One man had questions about his father who now has the early stages of the disease. And a woman was worried that her husband had the illness but he wouldn't discuss it. I don't think either one realized that hospice cares for people with Alzheimer's.

Alzheimer's is a disease that is appropriate for hospice care. In fact, to summarize the list of diseases and illnesses that are appropriate for hospice care is simple. Any disease that is chronic, meaning incurable, might be appropriate for hospice care when the patient's life expectancy is about six months due to the illness. Since Alzheimer's disease is chronic, hence incurable, when the doctor believes that the patient only has about six months of life remaining then, yes, calling hospice is appropriate.

It is paramount to remember that the following is a brief overview. It is up to a physician to determine how far the illness has progressed in a person.

So, how is it determined that a person has about six months of life remaining when they have Alzheimer's? A scale has been developed that charts a patient's decline in physical and mental abilities as the disease progresses. That scale is known as the F. A. S. T. Scale. These four letters stand for: Functional Assessment Staging Test. There are seven stages in this scale with Stage 7 being the one that indicates there may be only six months or less of life remaining.

Following is a brief generalization of the abilities of a person in each stage of the FAST scale:

Stage 1: Everything seems to be okay.

Stage 2: Forgetting names and losing objects becomes a problem.

Stage 3: Difficulty in traveling to new locations. Co-workers notice a decline in ability to perform job duties.

Stage 4: Decrease in ability to perform complex tasks such as planning dinner and handling finances.

Stage 5: Needs assistance in choosing proper clothing.

Stage 6: Increased difficulty in dressing, bathing, and using the bathroom until they cannot do these activities without assistance.

Stage 7: This is the stage in which a person becomes appropriate for hospice care. There are six areas of focus in this stage. They include:

SubStage 7a: Ability to speak is limited to approximately 1-5 words a day.

Sub   Stage 7b: All intelligible vocabulary is lost.

Sub   Stage 7c: Person is non-ambulatory, meaning that they cannot walk by themselves.

Sub   Stage 7d: Unable to sit up by themselves.

Sub Stage 7e: Unable to smile.
Sub Stage 7f: Unable to hold their head up.

Each person moves through the scale at their own pace. It is important to know that there may be a secondary medical problem which may complicate matters as far as the patient's abilities and their estimated life expectancy is concerned.

As mentioned, the above listing of the seven stages in the F.A.S.T. scale is a generalization. The attending physician would determine what stage on the scale an Alzheimer's patient is in, and in fact, if they are hospice appropriate.

Most illnesses can cause a physical and emotional strain on the caregiver, but a neurological illness such as dementia or Alzheimer's can be especially difficult. I hope that the information about the F.A.S.T. Scale will be of help to you if you are worried about a loved one.

Hospice is always available to offer help, and hope, to people who are facing a medical crisis. You are not alone.

~ What Kind of a Place is Hospice? ~

EVER WONDER WHAT kind of a place hospice is? Actually, hospice is not a place; it's a philosophy of care. Hospice is one of those ambiguous words that doesn't seem to have a definitive description. True, hospice is not a place, although there are hospice in-patient facilities such as The Pickering House in Lancaster, Ohio. Hospice is not one all-encompassing organization like the American Red Cross, although hospice care is available in every state in the Union, Washington D.C., and Puerto Rico.

A general definition is, "Hospice is an organization or program that provides, arranges, and advises on a wide range of medical and supportive services for dying patients and their family and friends" (Institute of Medicine, 1997). That definition seems so clinical for such a caring program but it does sum up what hospice does.

A hospice may be a for-profit hospice which is a business whose purpose is to make a profit, or it may be not-for-profit hospice, such as the hospice where I volunteer. The only purpose is to comfort patients and their families. A for-profit hospice may offer some services at reduced costs while the hospice where I volunteer offers all services related to the terminal illness at no cost.

What kind of a place is hospice? Now you know that it is not a place at all. Rather, it's a philosophy of care. You also now know that some hospices need to focus on making money while some hospices only want to comfort you and your family.

~ CAN'T BEAT THE PRICE ~

I SAW A cartoon in which a patient was sitting on the examining table and a doctor was holding a clipboard. The doctor says, "I guess we'll start by getting an X-ray of your wallet." That's what I felt like when I was in the middle of a two-year battle fighting a disease that included a few lengthy stays in the hospital. Even with insurance, the high deductibles made it a costly adventure for my family.

The medical needs of a patient are what most people think about when battling a serious illness. And, although many won't admit it, "How are we going to pay for all of this?" is a secondary, yet, troublesome concern. Having talked to quite a few people over the years about what brought them to the hospice where I volunteer, I found that many were hesitant because they thought that hospice would be expensive. And since in their eyes hospice is nothing but the next step of medical care along the way, the worry about how much it's going to cost comes up.

It's important to note that I am talking only about the hospice program I work for, FairHoPe Hospice and Palliative Care, Inc. We are a 501(c)(3) not-for-profit hospice and are not affiliated with any other hospice. Many hospices are not-for-profit as FairHoPe Hospice is, but some hospices are for-profit and, yes, they need to make money. My hospice, however, believes that making a profit shouldn't be a concern when caring for a person nearing the end of life.

One of the first things that lets people know many of their problems will be taken care of is that the minute they sign on to my hospice's compassion, all the expenses related to the terminal illness from that point forward, stop. What, no cost?! How does the hospice staff get paid? They always want to know what our angle is; we must get the money somehow.

The fact is any hospice receives its funds from several sources. Primarily, a hospice receives a large percentage of money for day-to-day operations from Medicare. In order to receive that reimbursement, the hospice must be Medicare certified. A hospice might also receive funds from Medicaid, should the person on service meet Medicaid's financial eligibility criteria.

Many of the people who come on hospice service have private health insurance policies with hospice coverage. I might add that my hospice will pay the deductible if there is one. Insurance coverage for hospice is becoming more prevalent as insurance companies have found that hospice care is much less costly than trying to fight a terminal illness at the end of life.

Any shortfall a hospice may incur from a lack of government or insurance support is recuperated through fundraisers and donations. Most local hospices present several fundraisers throughout the year. All hospices appreciate the support from the community for fundraisers. It seems that every community has charitable groups that put on fundraisers to benefit their local hospice. And many other charitable groups will have one-time events benefitting the local hospice. In addition, every local hospice is grateful for individual donations. Without all this community generosity, no hospice would be able to provide the extraordinary level of care to those they serve.

Another source of funding is from a variety of corporate gifts, grants from charitable organizations, and estates. As a side note, some hospices may also receive financial support from United Way designated for bereavement services, which many hospices provide at no cost. There are no public or government funds that I know of that are available to be used for bereavement.

Hospice is not just for the dying; we are also for the living. One hallmark of hospice is that we do everything possible to remove all the burdens that a serious illness creates, no matter how small, so that the patient and family can focus exclusively on each other. My hospice is there to help the patient and their family, not only to work their way through disease issues, but the financial issues, as well. We do not charge for our services; all our funds come from the above-mentioned sources.

The specialty of hospice care is total comfort. No one realizes the depth of comfort hospice provides until they call. When facing the unthinkable, think of hospice.

.

~ Making St. Peter Wait ~

WHEN PEOPLE SIGN on to hospice service soon enough, they tend to live longer than the doctor expected. There are many explanations and theories about that. I think that the core reason seems to be hospice care addresses "What ails you," as my mom would say. And in the last stage of life what ails you, believe it or not, may not be the illness. During the last stage of life what ails you is often in the spiritual and emotional realms, not the physical.

Hospice makes a concerted effort to hire those who we deem will connect with the ones we care for, i.e., view them as a person, not as a patient. That seems to make a lot of difference. When I'm talking to someone in the general public who has experienced hospice compassion, they immediately start talking about all the little things that the hospice staff did. I don't think many, if any, even mention the terminal condition. It is always a comment similar to, "the nurse became one of the family," or "the hospice aide was so gentle with Mom," or "the social worker talked to us as if we were some of their best friends."

I can just imagine when one of our patients reaches the Pearly Gates they'll see St Peter playing Solitaire. He'll ask them, "Where have you been? I've been expecting you." Their reply might be, "I'm sorry it took so long, but I was on hospice service."

If you don't mind making St. Peter wait, give hospice a call.

~ WHICH DOCTOR ~

MY MOM WAS loyal to her family doctor to the very end. I myself, trust my doctor above any other medical professional. (Although I still feel that I'm fairly well-versed in the art of self-diagnosis.) After all that they've been through with their doctor, some folks are hesitant to contact hospice. They don't want to lose contact with their doctor.

Well, did you know that with many hospices, including the one where I volunteer, you may retain your family doctor as your physician during this stage of your life? Your doctor would then become a part of your hospice team and would consult with the hospice doctor regarding your care

Or, if desired, hospice will care for the terminal illness while the family doctor continues to care for all the other medical problems. Just as there are specialists in cardiology, digestive illnesses, cancer, etc. hospice doctors are specialists in end-of-life care. Your doctor works with other specialists and he or she may work with us.

The third option is for the hospice doctor to assume care of the patient. In this case, the family doctor relinquishes responsibility for the patient's care. As with all situations involving patient care, hospice asks the question, "What does the patient want?" There is no specific rule as to which of the three scenarios to use.

Hospice is here to help and will work out a care plan that satisfies the patient. You won't have to worry about which doctor will be with you.

~ You Won't be Swept Away ~

ONE OF THE hesitations people have when considering calling hospice is the idea that once a person signs on to our service, they will be swept away, never to be seen again. Generally, the exact opposite happens if hospice is called soon enough. In particular, with my hospice the terminally ill person is "swept" back into life. And, depending upon the illness, the person is put back into as normal a life as possible.

Normally, during any sort of disease treatment or medical crisis, the person has to go somewhere, whether to a doctor's office, an Emergency Room or a clinic. Depending upon the severity of the illness, the person may be admitted to a hospital or nursing home. But with hospice, when we are called to help, we go to the patient. We will meet to discuss the situation wherever is convenient; whether in the home, a restaurant, or anywhere else. As much as is practical, we will care for the patient where they live. If the patient lives at home, they stay home. If they live in a house or apartment and need any special equipment, such as a hospital bed or oxygen, we bring it to them.

So, when someone signs on to hospice, they are not removed from life as they knew it before the illness struck. They are brought back, as much as possible, into the rhythm of life. Now that you know that you won't be swept away, consider hospice.

~ Your Bucket List ~

I MENTIONED TO a friend in conversation that I have driven through 47 States. I only had North Dakota left to go before I've driven in all 48 of the Continental United States.

"So, going to North Dakota is on your bucket list?" my friend asked.

"If I had a bucket list, I guess it would be," I replied. I really never thought about having such a list. I've been fortunate enough to do most of the things that I've wanted to do and to go to most of the places where I've wanted to go. For example, I didn't start out, as a youngster, wanting to drive through all 48 Continental United States. By my early 20's, I had made it to about half of them, so I decided to make it my goal get to all 50 states during my life. If nothing else, it was my goal to drive through all 48 of the continental United States. That plan, I guess you could say, became a part of my bucket list.

What is a bucket list, anyway? It's what is still known as a "wish list." Even though the term "bucket list" seems like it has been around for a long time, sociologists say that it's a recent term that has quickly woven itself into our language. It seems to be used most often by people in middle age who talk about things that they want to do before they die. The term is derived from one of the many euphemisms for dying, i.e.; "kick the bucket." So, a bucket list is a list of things that you want to do before you die or "kick the bucket."

The term really seems to have taken off after the movie, "The Bucket List," which came out in 2008. It starred Morgan Freeman and Jack Nicholson. They played two patients who were hospital roommates while receiving treatment for cancer in a hospital. Some of the movie critics didn't think that the movie was realistic. I agree with those critics who thought the movie was not true to life. My experience has been that there are few people diagnosed with terminal cancer who would have the energy to skydive, drive race cars or travel around the world.

What was true in the movie, though, is that family relationships dominated their conversation throughout their efforts to fulfill items on their list.

There are exceptions to every situation. Actually, the hospice where I volunteer did have a patient who had a bucket list, and skydiving was on his. He lived in a nursing facility and had enough stamina, mobility, and mental alertness to do it. So, the facility called my hospice and asked if we would allow one of our patients to skydive. The answer was a very fast "yes."

The patient, if I remember, was in his late 60's and it turned out to be a great event for the entire family. One of the Columbus TV stations interviewed the patient and put the event on the evening news.

My hospice does not sponsor any type of bucket list endeavor or special wish type of event. At the same time, we don't restrict our patients if they'd like to do something "they've always wanted to do," as in the case of the skydiving patient.

Our employees and volunteers, on their own initiative, have occasionally helped a patient, and their family, accomplish a desired goal. As mentioned previously, staff and volunteers have assisted our patients in going to the World War II Memorial in Washington D.C., to visit family in Mexico, and have gone to an oceanfront resort in Florida. In many of the parades that my hospice has participated in, one of the people on service rode with us. There will be more.

The real bucket lists, however, may not be so newsworthy. They may only include the simple things. We had a woman on service who wanted to ride in a helicopter. Some of our employees made a few phone calls and had the arrangements made for the ride. The pilot understood the situation and said that he would do whatever the patient wanted. He said he would fly her over her house or maybe just fly her around the airport. If she wasn't feeling too well on the day of the event the pilot said that he would just rise up 20' and come down, or just stay on the tarmac and rev up the engine. He was very considerate.

Most of the time a patient's bucket list is, indeed, very simple. Like in the Bucket List movie, the two main character's true bucket lists just dealt with family relationships. Jack Nicholson's character wanted to make amends with his grown daughter before he died.

Our chaplain was talking to a mother whose only wish was to hear her estranged daughter's voice. They had been apart for many years. The chaplain felt that the woman was holding on to life until she could hear her daughter's voice just once more. After a few phone calls from the chaplain and a little bit of coaxing, the daughter did call. That phone call, as you can imagine, meant everything to the mother.

I think that a lot of items on bucket lists could be accomplished if you just did it. Just go, if you've always wanted to go somewhere. Just sign up and take those dance lessons. Or call the county airport and tell them that you'd like to go skydiving. Do you realize that if you live within 450 miles of the ocean you can most likely go to the coast and come back over a weekend? Leaving on a Friday afternoon, it takes about 8 hrs. to travel 450 miles. Visiting the ocean during the off-season (no tourists) can be an unhurried, spiritual experience. Leaving the seashore at noon on Sunday, you should be home by 8 p.m.

I know that almost all of us plan to act upon the bucket list later or someday. If we decide to act when diagnosed as terminally ill, often it's too late for the simple reason that we are going to feel too sick or be too weak to even want to do anything. My observation has been that by the time someone is terminally ill, the wishes become one-more-time wishes – favorite meal one more time, sit out in backyard one more time, etc.

Take the time to reflect upon your life, where you've been and where you're going. If you've never thought about it, now may be the time to make your bucket list. A real bucket list should be accomplished while you're healthy and have energy. The list may help you put a focus back in your life and help you to focus on where you are going.

~ A Deer for the Deer Hunter ~

S EVERAL YEARS AGO, in late November, the hospice where I volunteer signed on a middle-aged man who was bitter that his life was being cut short. Linda, our full-time chaplain, talked to the man at length but could not determine what was at the root of his anger. She knew that maybe another man could relate to what was bothering the patient. Linda asked one of our part time chaplains, Charlie, if he would talk to the man. Charlie happened to be a retired Park Ranger.

After meeting the patient, Charlie quickly learned that the man was a deer hunter. He discovered that the patient was angry because his illness would prevent him from hunting this year and the State wouldn't bend the rules so that he could hunt one more time.

Through his connections with law enforcement (and, maybe God), Charlie was notified that a deer had just been hit by a car and he was permitted to remove it. He went home, put on his Ranger uniform, put the dead deer in the bed of his pickup and brought it to the hospice home where the man was briefly staying.

Although the temperature was November crisp, the chaplain rolled the patient's bed out to the parking lot so the patient could see and feel the deer. For the patient, it was a beautiful sight! His anger washed away. Charlie, in Park Ranger uniform, helped the patient to relive a part of his life and brought the man peace.

The people who work in hospice know it is of the utmost importance to give the people in our care peace and fulfillment at the end of life, no matter how simple it may seem.

~ A MOTHER'S LOVE ~

THIS EVENT WAS probably one of the most profound examples of the selflessness that is a mother's love that I've ever witnessed. I have said it before, that nowhere else will you see life at its most pure, basic intensity than in hospice.

I had been a volunteer for only a few years when my hospice accepted a young mother, "Sherry," on service. Up to that point, I had known Sherry casually because she was a regular customer at a charity bingo event where I also volunteered. She was always upbeat, attended the event with her family, and would only spend a small amount. For a period of several months she did not attend the weekly Friday event.

I soon found out that during those few months, Sherry was being treated for a very serious illness. The illness was being obnoxious and it wouldn't go away. After many tests and procedures, Sherry was told that her illness was terminal. That was the day before her 30th birthday.

When initially given the diagnosis, Sherry said that she was angry and felt that it wasn't fair. Understandably, since she was so young, all of Sherry's family and friends were adamant that she fight this and never give up. However, Sherry had some experience with hospice through a friend. She witnessed firsthand that hospice respected a family's right to make their own end-of-life decisions. She learned that hospice supports whatever decision is made. Sherry wanted to maintain control of her life for her daughter's sake, so she chose hospice.

And it was Sherry's only child, Mandi, who indirectly made the decision for her as to how she would spend the rest of life. Mandi was not quite a teenager and those difficult transitional teenage years were still ahead. Sherry's love for her daughter was a deep love, a mother's love, and she knew that for her daughter, she had to face reality. Confronted with the reality of what was happening, Sherry asked herself what was the most loving thing that she could do for her daughter. Instinctively, Sherry knew that as a mother she needed to be there for her daughter even if she couldn't be there.

Talking things over with her hospice social worker, Sherry learned that people have bought gifts to leave for their children to remember them after they have passed. Sherry liked that idea. She admitted that originally she didn't want to buy the gifts, thinking that if she didn't do it, then she wouldn't die. However, the symptoms from the illness told her that she had better get started.

These "future gifts" would remind her daughter that Mom would always be with her. Sherry spent several weeks buying cards and gifts. Her daughter was aware of the gifts, but didn't know what they were. Sherry wanted to store the gifts in something special so they went shopping together to buy a hope chest. Mandi picked out the one she liked.

Everything that Sherry purchased was wrapped in the appropriate gift-wrapping paper and went in the hope chest. She put post-it notes on the outside of everything so Mandi's dad would know what to give her at what time. And, as a backup plan, she wrote down each gift in a notebook.

Sherry bought gifts for all the important events in Mandi's life that she would miss. She bought a birthday card for her 21st birthday and wrote something in it for Mandi. Whether it was the Sweet 16 key chain to use for her car key when she got her driver's license or the bride and groom figurines for the top of her wedding cake, Mandi would know that her Mom was and always would be with her.

Sherry lived longer than expected. in part, I believe, because she had purpose. Her love for her daughter and her concern for Mandi, even when she was gone, was paramount in her life.

It is true that a mother's love is eternal. And, yes, some relationships between a mother and child can be strained, but a mother's love is always there – deep, abiding, unflinching. This intense love can make end-of-life decisions almost impossible to make, and at the same time, easier to make. A mother's love gives everything.

The end of life is not a medical event, it is a life event. Hospice assists its patients to live. It allows the patient to do what they need to do to make their life complete, to finish it the way they feel is necessary.

~ THOUGHTFUL, COMMITTED PEOPLE ~

I BEGAN MY career at the area hospice as a patient-contact volunteer back in the late 1990's. At that time, it consisted of approximately 30 paid employees and 30 volunteers. One of the things I noticed early on about our hospice was that if a person on service needed any kind of assistance, the staff was willing to help. It's hard to believe, but there were no cell phones. Yet we always responded to a crisis in short order. I was impressed that my hospice was definitely a small group of committed people.

An example of how we would respond happened on a Wednesday, early in my patient-contact volunteer career. The volunteer coordinator made a rare phone call to me at work. Usually she would call me in the evening so I figured that something was up. It was December 23 and my day job as a construction trailer leasing agent was slow. She asked if I would be interested in another patient assignment. Although I was visiting a patient on a regular basis, I never wanted, then or now, to say that I was too busy to help someone who was terminally ill. So, I agreed.

She gave me the usual information about the person I would be visiting: age, name of terminal disease, if any spouse and children, location, etc. Then she mentioned that I would have to drop in on them to work out a visiting schedule because their phone had been disconnected for nonpayment. She told me that the hospice social worker made arrangements for the phone to be reinstalled but it would take about two weeks. What? Two weeks and he's terminally ill? She said our social worker did what she could but because of the holidays, many of the linemen took time off and two weeks was the best that could be hoped for.

I knew that something had to be done about the phone situation. My problem was that I didn't know any "higher-ups" at the phone company who could pull strings. Besides, our social worker had tried everything. I happened to remember that the father of one of my son's friends, Mike, was a lineman for the phone company. I hoped that maybe he knew someone in management who could help. It took a little while to track down his wife who gave me Mike's mobile work number.

I called Mike, who was at a work site, and explained that a terminally ill man was going to have to possibly wait for two weeks before his phone was to be reconnected. This would cause tremendous communication problems and create more problems than already existed. He told me he was just "one of the grunts in the field" but would see what he could do.

In the meantime, there were several other issues that had to be dealt with because the family was poor. The dad, who was terminal and in his early thirties, had not been able to work for months. He had been the one with insurance. His wife, who made minimum wage and had no insurance, eventually quit her job to care for her husband. Looking at the situation from a distance, quitting her job wasn't the best idea, but they had no extended family to help and she did what she thought was best. Regardless, in any situation hospice staff doesn't look for fault; it's too late for that. We look for a remedy.

While the phone problem continued to be dealt with, the hospice staff was trying to arrange for the couple's three children to have a nice Christmas. But since this event happened so close to Christmas all the charitable organizations and groups having toy drives had given out their supply of toys. Undaunted, our six-member office staff took up a collection to buy the patient's children toys for Christmas. Two office staff hastily left for the mall.

The social worker, nurses and aides took up a collection among the medical staff and bought gift certificates to several stores with the idea that the parents could buy each other presents. Talking to the dad weeks later, he told me that those gift certificates were greatly appreciated by him and his wife because it allowed them to go shopping for their kids and not hand them donations on Christmas morning. That was vital for the parent's emotional well-being. They did not buy anything for each other.

Meanwhile, two hours after the call to the telephone lineman,

Mike, he called me back and simply said, "You've got a dial tone." Meaning the phone was reconnected. I was flabbergasted. I had to ask him to repeat it because I couldn't believe that he was able to cut the time down from two weeks to less than two hours. He was very modest about it and explained that as each job request, or "work order" comes in, it's placed at the end of the list. The linemen are to take each work order at the front of the list, not pick and choose. Mike said that there was no question about what had to be done so he did it. Personally, I think that this was a classic case of the last shall be first.

The joy of brightening that family's life was truly the joy of Christmas for the hospice staff and volunteers who spontaneously bore the weight of the burden and changed a bleak Christmas into one of love. Christmas in its purest form is when you celebrate it by giving love to those who need it most.

All things considered, Christmas for the family of five turned out just fine. They had a small Christmas tree set up in the living room, toys under the tree and presents *bought by mom and dad.* And they had a phone to call their friends at hospice if they needed anything. Anthropologist Margaret Mead once said, "Never doubt that a small group of thoughtful, committed people can change the world; indeed, it is the only thing that ever has."

~ A Wonderful Fall Wedding ~

IT'S BEEN said that death comes either too soon or too late. And our society has been trying to make sure it doesn't come too soon. Fighting to the bitter end and doing whatever it takes to get one more day seems to be everyone's goal. But at what price? The hospice where I volunteer allows life to go on as normal as possible, like natural childbirth but on the other end. It's amazing, no –make that profound – what can happen when we allow life to happen as it should.

In my hospice's case, we keep the person at home and involved with life (if their health allows) even though the end may seem imminent. My hospice's purpose is to assist…not speed up or slow down the natural rhythm of life. The following story, which happened several years ago, is a nice way to show how we are focused on our patient's life, not their illness.

Several years ago, in the Spring, a young woman became engaged. What a joy for her mom – so many things to do. It was exciting as mother and daughter planned the wedding. The mom, Jen, reminisced about when she was planning her own wedding with her mom. As June arrived, plans were in full swing and the Fall wedding was in sight. However, by early July, Mom was tiring very easily. After several doctor visits, the mom broke the news to her daughter that she had Stage IV cancer. The cancer seemed to be growing rapidly and the doctor estimated that she only had a few months of life remaining.

The daughter, though stunned, immediately decided to postpone her wedding, allowing everyone to focus on her mother. She felt that her mom's situation was much more urgent and important than the wedding. Jen absolutely refused, though, reasoning that her life was coming to an end but that her daughter's was just beginning. Each tried to put the other first. The daughter relented and kept the wedding date as planned. The family knew of hospice's compassion so Jen was placed on service. This allowed her to be cared for at home and to continue helping with the wedding preparations.

As the September days went by, Jen's pain level increased. Concern grew that she would not be able to attend the wedding. Or worse, that she might not live to see her daughter's wedding. With less than ten days until the wedding, Jen was brought to my hospice's facility, The Pickering House, for one of its main purposes, symptom management. In this case the symptom was pain. The Pickering House's staff carefully brought Jen's pain down to a tolerable level while keeping her fully aware of her surroundings, very important if she were to watch her little girl walk down the aisle.

Probably the most important duty of a mother on her daughter's wedding day is to be nearby when needed. And Jen was. Her "home-side" nurse, Katy, spent the night before at the family's home and accompanied her to the church, even assisting with getting Jen ready. Everyone could now focus on the day knowing that medical assistance was right there. Katy sat with the congregation as the Wedding March began. All eyes turned toward the back and were startled to see three people begin the walk down the aisle. With sniffles accompanying the music, Jen was escorted on one side by her daughter, the bride, and on the other side by her brother. I think that even the church mouse had a tear in his eye as the three slowly approached the altar. She had done it!

The hospice nurse, Katy, sat with Jen during the ceremony. Too tired for the reception, Jen laid down in a room prepared by Katy. She rested and said that she needed to talk to her dad who was already in Heaven. Even the wedding photographer did what he could to help by working over the weekend, preparing all the photos so that Mom could enjoy them at The Pickering House on Monday. On Wednesday, Jen went to be with her dad.

Hospice is in the life business. We allow life to go on as it should, including wonderful Fall weddings.

~ Basic Nursing ~

THE TERM "NURSE" is one of those career descriptions that, as the field expands and adds more responsibilities, seems to be getting less clear cut about what that career entails. I think that the simplest definition of a nurse is, "A person trained to care for the sick and infirm." On the other side of the coin, The American Nursing Association states, "Nursing is the protection, promotion, and optimization of health and abilities, prevention of illness and injury, alleviation of suffering through diagnosis and treatment of human response, and advocacy in the care of individuals, families, communities, and populations."

Not too long ago, my hospice received a Thank You card from a man whose wife had died on our service. In it, he thanked "...the nurse who sat on the floor at (my wife's) bedside with us when she had expired. (The nurse) waited patiently and lifted our spirits while waiting for the funeral director to arrive to retrieve the body." The woman had died at home and there were no chairs in the bedroom. No one wanted to leave her alone, so they sat on the floor. That is what my hospice's nurses do. I've heard it said that, "People don't care how much you know until they know how much you care."

There is absolutely a need for advanced degreed nurses, nursing professors, directors, leaders, etc. But at the end of life, the only need is for "A person trained to care for the sick and the infirm," a hospice nurse.

~ Bob's Unforgettable Dance ~

BOB HAD BEEN a hospice patient for a while. He lived at home but it became necessary to bring him to The Pickering House (our hospice facility) for some extra care. He'd been there before. The first time he came he drove himself to The House so that he could leave if he didn't like it. Now he likes to joke that he had to be evicted that first time. "It's a good place."

Gayle, one of our volunteers and an accomplished singer, decided to stop in and visit Bob one evening during this most recent stay. Several of Bob's family members were there and realized that they were in for an unexpected treat. The mood was perfect as only one lamp was lit in Bob's room.

Gayle sang a few '50's love songs to Bob. Listening to her, Bob was reminded of the dances in high school. "You've got me in the mood for dancing," he exclaimed in an almost giddy voice. Well, that's all it took. Gayle extended her hand, he accepted and stood up. At first it was a slow dance at arm's length. As Gayle began to softly sing the song, "Unforgettable," Bob drew Gayle close. They were soon slowly swaying cheek to cheek as she sang in almost a whisper. There wasn't a dry eye in the house. His niece took a picture. The serene, heavenly look on Bob's face, in that picture, is the one that's worth those thousand words we've all heard about.

"Unforgettable, in every way. And forevermore, that's how you'll stay."

~ CELEBRATE THE LASTS ~

ANYONE WORKING OR volunteering at a hospice knows that we celebrate life. We celebrate life and help our patients and their families celebrate life. One of the ways we do this is to recognize the last moments of life and help people celebrate those occurrences. In only a short while after becoming a volunteer, I realized that one of the honors of being a patient care volunteer is the fact that most likely the volunteer is the last "new" person that the patient will ever meet. I had not thought about that but it's probably true.

I got to thinking about how many people I have met in my life and how many more I have yet to meet. And by this, I mean either formally introduced, or interacted with in some capacity. How many people does an ordinary person meet during their entire life; 15,000, 30,000? Studies have estimated (guessed?) that we may have had contact with as many as 120,000 people during our lifetime.

It has been said that time decides who you meet in life, your heart decides who you want in your life, and your behavior decides who stays in your life. So, I guess a variation of that question would be to ask, "How many people will you have an impact on during your life?"

When you think about it, starting at birth you are (sort of) introduced to your mother and father, then immediate family, then aunts and uncles, cousins, and gradually to friends, teachers, clergy, coaches, spouse(s), in-laws, coworkers, neighbors, and medical personnel. And finally, should you choose hospice, you meet your hospice team. The volunteer is usually the last person on the team that the patient will meet. I try to treat everyone I am introduced to as the last person he will ever meet and to be honored by it. That seems to emphasize the importance of "lasts" as much as "firsts."

Our society celebrates the firsts in life but it usually doesn't celebrate the lasts. We celebrate baby' first word but what about the last word uttered before death? We celebrate baby's first step but when was the last step taken, as an adult, before he couldn't get out of bed anymore? We celebrate the first time that baby put the spoon in her mouth all by herself, but when was the last time she fed herself before illness left her too weak to lift the spoon?

Personally, I remember the thrill that I experienced the first time, as a little boy when I broke away from my Dad, running alongside me, and rode a two-wheeler by myself. But when did I park my bike in the garage, as a teenager, for the last time? That, also, was a milestone and one of those subtle transitions from childhood to adulthood. And when was the last time I played Hide and Seek with my friends in the neighborhood? Although I must admit that I do remember leaving high school on the last day as a senior and celebrating that "last" life event.

Life has as many lasts as it does firsts. We rarely celebrate the lasts because we rarely know when they occur. The hospice staff is aware of how the body slowly turns itself off during the last stage of life and lets a family member know when such a subtle event has begun. It can be profound.

In another instance a husband and wife, with the help of hospice staff and volunteers, were able to celebrate their 58th, and last, wedding anniversary at home surrounded by their family just hours before the husband died. In a third example, the hospice staff was able to help a son and his dad go fishing together one last time before the dad died.

When people who are not familiar with it hear the word "hospice," they think of sadness. They don't think for a minute that there can be time to be happy and to celebrate. Yes, there can be. In early life, you celebrated the firsts. In later life, hospice helps you to complete the circle of life and celebrate the lasts. We consider it an honor to be the last few people that a patient will meet on this Earth, and we try to make them the best.

~ This Night Was Different ~

"**D**ATE NIGHT IS one of the most important appointments on this busy Mama's calendar," according to happily married Lisa. She was discussing what she knew was a necessity to having a happy marriage. And that is, having one night every month in which she and her husband took time for themselves. On Date Night, the babysitter arrives as scheduled, fixes dinner, reads stories, and plays with the children. The babysitter then tucks the kids in bed and stays as late as necessary in order to give Lisa time to go on a date with her "Sweetheart of 17 years," husband Rob. Lisa says that, "Our babysitter, Sarah, is worth every penny we pay her." The couple always comes home feeling refreshed and renewed in their love for one another.

Activities on Date Night may involve any fun activity that comes to mind. They may go off to the bike trail, or to dinner, a movie, or to shop (Wow, it must be love!) It's an experience that is treasured when raising five little ones.

Their latest Date Night was a bit different than the many others they've had over the years. Lisa and her husband agreed that this particular night was made richer and sweeter for the way it began. They planned to start the night by making a short stop to visit someone whom they'd recently met. That short stop, however, turned into a very fulfilling evening.

Instead of going to a dinner or a movie they stopped by the hospice facility to visit the patient to whom Lisa had recently been assigned. The couple, in fact, are hospice patient contact volunteers. In its volunteer ranks the hospice where they volunteer has more than a few couples who volunteer together. Lisa and Rob visited her patient, "Jim," who was staying at the hospice in-patient facility while his caregivers took a much-needed respite (i.e., rest) from their full-time care of him.

For this Date Night, the couple visited Jim, talked with him, laughed with him, and sat quietly with him. The greatest gift you can give someone is your full attention and Lisa's husband listened intently as Jim talked about his life in construction. It was so important for Jim to tell someone about his life and his accomplishments. He needed to celebrate his life with someone. As Lisa related, "He needed his back scratched and a listening ear, and we were there."

Later that evening when the couple left, they realized the blessings of sharing their precious alone time with Jim. Lisa said that, "It gave us perspective on how brief our lives are here on Earth. How in giving of ourselves we receive and how very real is the need for fellowship with others in our life's journey. We thank God for the opportunity to briefly share in Jim's time at the facility." Lisa confided later that she saw tenderness in Rob that she had never seen before and she felt a deeper closeness to him. The couple agreed that by thinking of another before themselves, this Date Night turned out to be their best one.

~ Dogs Just Know ~

MY EXPERIENCE WITH dogs is that they seem to immediately know who is good, or safe, and who isn't. One theory I've heard is that possibly dogs can see an aura around us and that helps them to know, by the color of the aura, if the person is good or not. That's probably theory more than scientifically proven fact but anyone who owns a dog knows to take the "advice" of a dog about whom to trust.

A volunteer tells of his experience with a Dachshund named Oscar who, to a degree, proved the aura theory. When the volunteer arrived at a new patient's home for his first visit, the wife answered the door after he rang the doorbell. "You're from hospice, aren't you? I knew when you pulled up on the driveway that you were from hospice," she said. (I might note that at that time our hospice staff wore very small black badges with white letters.)

She went on to tell the volunteer that Oscar feels that it's his duty to bark when anyone pulls into the driveway, even family members. He will bark again when they ring the doorbell. Yet for some reason Oscar would silently run to the door and sit patiently when any hospice staff or volunteer arrived. What defied explanation is that the person, such as the volunteer, may never have been there before. Yet Oscar never barked.

You may be apprehensive about trusting someone unfamiliar into your house when a family member is ill. Don't worry, hospice staff and volunteers seem to be good, and safe. Just ask your dog.

~ Cats May Not Seem Interested ~

I THINK IN every area of healthcare the paramount focus of the medical staff is the illness. And it has to be that way. The only reason anyone goes to a healthcare professional is, well, for health. During your office visit, the healthcare professional may ask a few questions about your family but it's usually just idle chatter or to ask who will drive you home after a treatment. And they generally don't include your pet in your care plan. With our healthcare system the way it is, there is only time to focus on the illness.

People consider hospice to be the last stage of the health care continuum. The last house on the block, so to speak. We're not. The last specialist that you visited is actually your last stop on the healthcare continuum. The focus of hospice is completely different than a normal doctor's focus. Hospice does not focus on the illness, but rather, it focuses on the patient who is ill. Not only does hospice focus on the person but on every part of the patient's life; family, friends, home life, spiritual life, and pets.

Pets? Do we give some of our attention to the person's pets when the ill person is in their last stage of life? Yes, we do. Not only do we notice the pets, but we understand that we must pay attention to them. They often help us if we watch and listen. In one particular instance, a hospice patient had an indoor cat. As a person with a cat, I know that there are no ordinary cats. This cat soon proved that he was a smart cat even though, like the typical unassuming cat, he never let on that he was interested in anything but sleeping.

A family member told me of his last visit with this patient. The patient was being cared for in his home and had his bed set up in the living room. The patient liked to be a part of the action and didn't want to be sequestered back in his bedroom so his bed was placed where the couch had been.

On this particular evening, family had gathered at the house because the patient's health was declining at a noticeable rate. The patient became tired, so family and friends, who had gathered, moved to the kitchen to allow him to rest quietly. About 20 minutes later the conversation in the kitchen was suddenly interrupted by the patient's cat. It came running into the kitchen from the living room and, as one of the family members put it, "Just threw a fit. There's no other way to describe it; he just threw a fit." At first no one could figure out what was wrong with the cat but someone suggested that they check on the patient.

Very quickly they noticed that the patient's breathing pattern had changed. This was not a good indication. Months earlier, when the patient signed on to hospice care, the nurse explained to the family certain things that may happen as the body begins the normally slow process of turning itself off. After they went to the patient's bedside they realized that he had begun the Cheyne-Stokes (pronounced "chain stokes") breathing that signals the end is near.

The family called hospice to let them know what was going on. Then they pulled up chairs around the bed and sat in silent prayer. In less than an hour, the patient died. Now they understood that the cat sensed the end was very close and was trying to get everyone's attention.

As I've mentioned the focus of hospice is not on the illness but on the person. Hospice includes the family pet in the patient's care plan since pets are a part of the family. Cats may not seem interested but they may become a little more involved than expected, as this cat did. And that is fine with us because hospice knows that even a cat might help.

~ Graduating from Hospice ~

I VOLUNTEERED AT a charitable weekly bingo game a few years ago. It was a lot of fun because we had such a great group of regular customers. I got to know quite a few of them. One customer in particular was a man in his early thirties. To make a long story short, he stopped coming to the bingo game and within a few months signed on to hospice compassion. I was shocked because, in my opinion, he was just too young to be on our service. Since he knew me he requested that I visit him as his hospice volunteer, and bring him a few instant win "goldies."

He was one of the fortunate people who signed on to hospice soon after being given a terminal diagnosis. By doing so, hospice had plenty of time to comfort him and his family. And, as what may happen when someone signs on soon enough, his health improved. He was no longer appropriate for hospice care.

When someone's health improves to the point that they no longer qualify for hospice service they are revoked – meaning that the patient is dismissed from our service. We refer to that as "graduating" from hospice. From my perspective, if I'm going to graduate from anything, I'd like to graduate from hospice.

As a footnote, I saw him at last year's Fourth of July parade, 14 years after he "graduated."

~ It is of Absolute Importance ~

UNTIL AROUND 50 years ago, death tended to be sudden. If not sudden, then death came relatively quickly following a terminal diagnosis. Today, with progress in medical technology and the development of new treatments, the dying process is being transformed into a lengthy ordeal. And if the illness allows, the care may be given in the comforting confines of home.

In a family, care giving at home is a job that was not always asked for, but a job of absolute importance. Eventually it may become just that – a job. Although we may admire caregivers and even look at their tasks as a sacred duty, care giving to a family member at home can be a lonely task and a physically demanding one. No matter how necessary the job is or how lovingly it's done, after a while even the strongest relationship will become strained and need some help. Over time stress and tensions will emerge. That, along with managing their life outside of the caregiving role creates additional stress on the caregiver.

When a family member receives a disease prognosis of six months or less, consider asking hospice for assistance. Our purpose is to assist and comfort both the patient and the family. I have found it's quite common for hospice to put as much effort into comforting the caregiver and their family as in comforting the patient. By assisting a family, hospice allows them to focus on what is of absolute importance; their relationship with the terminally ill family member. Granted, caregiving is important but what is of absolute importance are family relationships.

~ ALL IN THE FAMILY ~

I ARRIVED FOR my first visit with the new patient at 6 pm. The patient, a man in his 30's, had moved back home so that his parents could care for him during his last stage of life. Serious illness in a family has a way of upsetting the daily routine of life, creating upheaval, and quite often a shortening of tempers. And that was the situation in this household.

One of the family's routines that I learned was that the four-legged member of the family, a Schnauzer named Schultz, liked to be let out for his evening constitutional at 7 pm. As the parents were preparing to leave for dinner, and to get a little reprieve from the constant care giving, the man leaned down and told the dog to sit. He told Schutz to remind me to let him out at 7 pm. "At seven on the dot, do you understand?" he said firmly to the dog. Schultz gave a one bark affirmative answer.

Sure enough, at seven on the dot, Schultz barked once, then went to the back door. Maybe it was his German heritage, but Schultz liked things done as they should be, and when they should be. Over the next few months I learned that if I didn't get there soon enough, he'd bark again.

A serious illness can upset everyone's schedule. Hospice will do what it can to maintain the stability of routine in the life of the person who is ill and their family. Even the four-legged members of the house.

~ Everyone Affected ~

DO YOU REALIZE that hospice compassion benefits everyone affected by a serious illness? And by everyone, I'm including the spouse, siblings, parents, children, grandparents, grandchildren, nephews, nieces, in-laws, friends, and pets. Even the cat, if it's interested.

When someone in the family has a very serious illness, everyone wants to fight it to the bitter end. Hospice understands that and it respects anyone's desire to fight to the end. My experience has shown me that the hospice way is calm, serene, with family and friends nearby being supported by our staff and volunteers. But honestly, I don't think anyone knows what decision they'll make until they arrive at that juncture. I've found that serenity always comes when you stop expecting miracles and start accepting life on life's terms.

Sometimes, no matter how close a family is, it can come apart under the stress of every hour of every day of every week of every month of caring for someone. A spouse may no longer feel like a spouse but rather like an overworked caregiver. Children, whether younger or in adulthood, may become resentful if they feel that none of their siblings are helping. There are a myriad of situations and family dynamics that arise when someone enters the last stage of life.

If you're caring for someone in your home and feel like you've just had enough, call hospice. Don't let your overdoing be your undoing. We have a lot of experience in caring for people in the last stage of life. Everyone affected by the terminal illness will be comforted.

~ Hospice Nurse ~

I AM CONSTANTLY impressed by what I hear when I talk to any of my hospice's amazing nurses. What they do is inspiring, yet many times they just perform simple gestures. What makes it possible for the nurses to do their work every day is that they are not afraid of the pain: the physical pain, the emotional pain, the spiritual pain. They are not afraid to feel it, nor are they afraid to be with a family member who is hurting. Some of our nurses have said that because they are not afraid, the caregiver's hurting seems to be lessened a bit.

A while ago, I was talking to one of our nurses, Mary. During our conversation, we talked about a home visit that she had just returned from. She casually mentioned that as she was preparing to leave, the patient's wife seemed to be at her wit's end. Mary asked her what the problem was and she explained her frustration in not being able to do everything she felt she was expected to do in caring for her husband. Mary knew that the woman had had enough.

Mary offered to stay and sit with the patient while his wife rested. Although taken back by the offer, the woman laid on the couch while Mary sat at the bedside of the patient and did paperwork. The unanticipated two-hour nap made all the difference in the world. Mary said, "As a hospice nurse, I simply do what is needed, and that was needed."

Hospice nurses are amazing people.

~ Importance of Food ~

SOMETHING THAT YOU don't hear mentioned very often when discussing hospice is food. Are you kidding? Food at a time like this?! Food is probably the last thing that comes to mind when someone you know is extremely ill. The obvious reason you wouldn't think of discussing food in the hospice setting is because the purpose of food is to sustain life. It's central to life.

What we eat sustains both the physical aspects of life, i.e., our bodies, and it sustains the emotional aspects of life. Think of eating pizza while watching The Rose Bowl on TV. Pizza is more for the emotional side than the nutritional side. Since the hospice where I volunteer celebrates life, it makes sense that food is an important part of what we do.

The truth is, food plays a role in our emotional health as well as our nutritional health. It can create a bridge to our past, just like music and photographs do. Eating is at the heart of all our celebrations and important events in life. Each of the holidays has special food associated with them. For example: ham at Easter, Thanksgiving turkey and fixings, hamburgers, and hot dogs on the grill for the summer holidays, etc.

One of the conveniences for the families of a patient having a short stay at our hospice house is the family kitchen. The kitchen allows families to fix their own meals if they would like, thus helping them to maintain some normalcy in their life. The kitchen contains a conventional oven, microwave, sink, refrigerator, dish washer, coffee maker, pots and pans, silverware, and bowls, plates, glasses, cups and serving dishes. It's complete. All the family has to do is bring in the groceries to prepare their own food. For a family in crisis, the activity of cooking can be therapy in itself.

As an example, a patient was brought in to the hospice house to give his wife a break from the constant activity of caring for him. He told our Kitchen Manager that his favorite meal was Thanksgiving dinner, but since it was August he was resigned to the fact that he will never have that feast again. He didn't realize how our staff listens and responds to such lamenting. He mentioned that the best part of the meal was his son-in-law's homemade noodles. For our hospice house staff that's all it took. The decision was made to have Thanksgiving dinner the next day. What, Thanksgiving dinner in August!? Why not?

Phone calls were made to the family, especially the son-in-law, and plans were made. The next morning family started arriving at the house. The hospice house's family kitchen was a hive of activity as the son-in-law rolled out the dough to make the noodles and the turkey was in the roaster. Staff brought in a long table and placed a linen table cloth on it. The patient's grandkids set the table, the balance of the dinner was prepared and by afternoon everything was ready.

The patient's bed was rolled to the head of the table so that, with help, he could carve the turkey. Having the man of the house carve the turkey was an endearing tradition in this family. All the effort put forth by the family and the hospice house staff demonstrated the emotional importance of food and the rituals that go with it.

That was by no means the only instance in which our caring staff knew just what the patient and family needed. During a conversation with Linda, our Kitchen Manager, I asked her how she could know our patients and their families so well, and in such a short time. She said that when she begins her shift, she'll visit each patient in order to find out a little bit about them. She'll ask about their favorite food and how they like it prepared. Always during the conversation, talking about food sparks memories of holidays, parties, and even cooking blunders.

Since Linda always has time for our patients, she'll listen. As she listens, she learns about family traditions, funny cooking mistakes, and memories of making cookies with Grandma when they were young. In essence, Linda helps the patient to accomplish a very important aspect of hospice. And that is, for the patient to recount important memories of their life. One woman told the story of her first pumpkin pie she baked with a top crust. After all those years it was still a favorite family story.

Another way in which food helps the patient emotionally is, should they come to the hospice house for a few days' stay, the cook will come to the patient's room and ask them what they'd like and how they want it fixed. We don't operate strictly off a menu. The importance of this is that in many instances the patient has been on diet restrictions and hasn't been able to order what they want, let alone eat it. Now they get to ask for whatever they want and it will be brought to their room. There are instances where everyone involved knew that the patient couldn't eat what they ordered because of an inability to chew, or some other reason, but it was nonetheless brought to them. They ordered it and received it and that is what was important. If what they want isn't on hand, the cook will go grocery shopping to get it. And as Linda says, "We even have real mashed potatoes. I peel and mash them myself."

Many times, a patient will return to the hospice house in about a month to give their caregivers another break. For this return visit, the cook will have all their favorite food ready to prepare should the patient want what they had on their previous visit. One patient, upon his second stay, had his stack of three pancakes, with a pat of butter between each pancake, brought in for his breakfast without even asking. Seeing this amount of attention shown to him, his wife was brought to tears.

These simple acts of love by our staff show that hospice understands the importance of food in the last stage of life. This focus on food lets the patient know that they are alive and still part of society. It gives them a sense of self-respect and the feeling that they still have control over their life. Food, at a time like this, is another way that hospice focuses on celebrating the life of its patients.

~ THE FAMILY'S PERSPECTIVE ~

THE HOSPICE WHERE I volunteer sets up displays in each of the county fairs in its three-county service area. When someone who has experienced the compassion of hospice sees the display, they want to stop by and say thanks. One of the nice things about representing a hospice at a county fair is that I get to hear about the great hospice efforts from the family's perspective. People who have "been there, got the t-shirt" so to speak.

People will come up to our display and thank the hospice representative who is there. They'll express their gratitude for the understanding and empathy extended to them, their family, and especially their loved one. In one instance, I was at the Hocking County Fair at our display in the Art Hall when a woman, whom I'll refer to as "Sarah" came up to thank me. She was grateful for hospice helping her mom, but made it a point to tell me that we also helped the entire family. Her mom had been on our service six years ago, but Sarah could remember everything as if it occurred last week.

Sarah began the conversation by saying that she had no previous experience with hospice. That used to be a common statement. Thankfully, we hear that less frequently as more and more people experience the goodness of hospice. Because of Sarah's lack of personal experience and only hearing comments here and there about hospice, she was very apprehensive when she made the call to us.

Sarah was amazed by our attention not only to her mom but to the family, as well. Sarah added that her mom's nurse was truly an angel. What this daughter noticed, and felt, was a calmness and empathy from the nurse. Sarah said that the nurse did nothing dramatic or newsworthy. The little, almost unnoticeable, things the nurse did was what impressed Sarah. Things like freely giving her time to the family. And "time" is a theme that comes through in so many of the compliments we receive.

In this case, Sarah said that the nurse took the time to teach her and her siblings special techniques in caring for their mom that the terminal illness dictates. She also said that the nurse "gave of her time to tell me and my family about other families' situations so that we knew we weren't alone. What we were feeling: scared, overwhelmed, and exhausted, was normal." Sarah said that the nurse took the time to educate them about the different stages of her mom's illness so that they would know what to look for and what to expect.

Sarah described how the nurse would sit and talk to her Mom. "The nurse got to know Mom so that she knew how to recognize when Mom was feeling stress." And that was not all. According to Sarah, "The nurse even went to Mom's calling hours after she died." ("Calling Hours are sometimes known as the "Visitation" at a funeral. It's where friends and family gather, usually at the funeral home, to talk to the family of the deceased.) She was so impressed that our nurse took the time out of her busy schedule to do that. "I just never expected that level of love," Sarah told me. I might add that last comment is heard quite often when talking about hospice care.

The daughter went on to tell me that hospice's entire staff displayed that level of empathy. She said the home health aide who came to help with her mom's care calmly, patiently taught them how to bathe her mother in such a way that it wouldn't cause mom any discomfort. The daughter said, "Because of Mom's disease, sometimes it was hard to move her without causing her pain."

She described our aide as another hospice angel who took as much time as they needed to advise them in caring for their mom and to comfort them too. The aide did what was needed. On one particular visit, her mom was not feeling well enough to be bathed, so the aide didn't bathe her. It was just that simple. But she stayed and talked to the family. As Sarah said, "She wasn't task oriented, she was *us* oriented."

Sarah went on to tell me how one night her mom couldn't sleep because of the symptoms of her disease. Sarah related how she called the night duty nurse. The night nurse could have given Sarah instructions over the phone but, instead, chose to drive out to their house in the middle of the night to take care of it himself. (We also have male nurses.) He wanted to make sure that the medicine would make the mom comfortable. Sarah told me, "He sat at her bedside. Occasionally he'd tell us that mom was doing much better."

In another example, and at a different fair, I talked to a woman about the great service we give to families and their loved ones. She concurred with what I was saying because we had cared for her father several months earlier. Then she sort of caught me off guard by telling me that the one thing that really impressed her about hospice was that we "weren't there when we weren't needed." I stepped back and had to think about that for a minute.

She told me that her dad was being cared for in her home. After about four weeks, hospice brought him into their facility in order to give the family a little break from the care giving. She said that one evening she and her siblings "were getting Daddy ready for bed. The door to the room was closed and as we were busy getting him ready, the door slowly opened. The nurse came in a few feet and stopped. She stood there for a few minutes, then gave me a thumbs up and left."

The woman told me that she didn't know what the nurse wanted but she knew that for her family, taking care of her dad was the most important thing. "She just left us alone." This woman went on to say that in other situations the hospice house staff "... only became involved if needed. If we were taking care of Daddy the way we wanted to, they just left us alone."

No matter what you think you know about hospice, if you ever find yourself in a situation where calling may be one of the options, ask your friends if they have hospice experience. Don't take our word for what we do – try to hear it from the family's perspective.

~ Good-byes are Necessary ~

WE SAY IT all the time – *Bye, Have a nice day! Later, dude! See you tomorrow. So long for now, TTYL!* Yet, we really don't think very much about it, do we? But what if it were the last good-bye, the final farewell with your loved one? As a family gathers at the bedside of a loved one who is dying, they often ask: "What do we do? What do we say?"

I have found that most people have a desire to say those final farewells. Yet many hesitate to say good-bye. One reason some people hesitate is that they think it will seem as though they have given up hope of the person being healed. Some hesitate because they fear that saying those final farewells might speed up their loved one's death. And some just don't know what to say. The truth is that when the time comes, you will say what needs to be said.

Yes, good-byes are necessary and are one of the advantages of hospice care. We give you the time and privacy to say what needs to be said. Don't hesitate to tell your loved one how much you love them and how greatly they will be missed. They need to know how special they were in your life. Tell them that you will be okay.

Saying good-bye is better said sooner than later. Talking to them while they are still coherent may open up a dialogue to discuss what needs to be said. If you say good-bye and the Lord gives you more time with your loved one, what have you lost? You have gained another opportunity to tell them how important they still are to you. Maybe some of these things should be said to others while there is plenty of time.

~ Hospice is a Life Sentence ~

HOSPICE IS A life sentence! That sounds like an oxymoron until you understand what we do at hospice. The truth is, when someone enters the last stage of life, each day becomes more intense, more precious. So, let's enjoy it, if the illness allows, rather than suffering the after-effects of one more treatment that may not actually extend life.

Much of the work of my hospice is not medical related. Hospice comforts physical pain, emotional pain, and spiritual pain. All three areas are equally important at the end of life. When someone accepts hospice, the ill person's care team concentrates on removing each area of pain, at which point, life becomes a precious gift to both the patient and their family.

Besides "normal" care, hospice offers many therapies to enhance one's life. Therapies include massage therapy, pet therapy, and music therapy. I was recently at a funeral service in which our Music Therapist, Erin, talked to those in attendance. She mentioned how the deceased person had taught her his favorite old hymn, one of the few hymns that she was not familiar with. Erin related that she now sings this hymn to other patients, thus carrying on the man's legacy. What a comfort it was for his family to hear that even in the last weeks of the man's life he had a positive influence on someone.

Hospice allows people to live pain free and to still have purpose during the last stage of life. Yes, hospice is a life sentence.

~ Look at All Sides ~

WHEN TOLD THAT she would be doing part of her clinicals at a hospice, the nursing student wasn't too thrilled. She said when she first found out where her assignment would be many thoughts ran through her mind, and none of them were good. "Am I only going to be around old people? Are they all bedridden? Do they have dementia? Can they still talk?" She realized that all her thoughts about hospice were negative. She had to admit that her initial thought of hospice was that it would be a depressing place. After all, don't people go there to die? She had a case of "Contempt without Investigation."

But as she accompanied the hospice nurse on her rounds, the student became involved in what hospice does and her impression of hospice changed completely. The first thing she learned about hospice, at least this hospice, was that people don't go there; hospice comes to them. In her own words, she said that, "I have come to realize I have never been more wrong about anything."

That response has universally been my experience after talking to someone who has been involved with hospice. After an experience with hospice, "If only I knew," is the common comment I hear from many of the ill person's family members.

As a whole, society's way of thinking about the end of life is changing just as our intern's did. The idea of making the act of dying a medical experience is only decades old. In his best selling book entitled, "*Being Mortal*" Dr. Atul Gawande (2014) stated, "As recently as 1945 most deaths occurred in the home. By the 1980's just 17% did." Dying had become viewed as a medical event and was no longer thought of as a natural or spiritual event. The view of dying came to be viewed as something that happened in an institution;. mainly at a hospital or nursing home.

And that way of thinking, that death was a medical event, was held by society as a whole. Both doctors and the family of a patient seemed to feel that for a seriously ill person, everything possible should be done to prolong life. The thinking was that everyone will die eventually, but don't let them die now. Actually, that still seems to be the way most people look at things when involved with an end-of-life crisis.

The steady growth of hospice care seems to indicate that the general public is starting to understand how hospice care can be a tremendous comfort. But the medical field, with encouragement from families, often remains focused on the pursuit of longevity of life no matter what. Not much thought is given to good quality of life. Quality of life is what hospice is about, and that is where the basic conflict lies.

The hospice where I volunteer allows the people on its service to pursue their dreams and to have priorities other than just to live longer. Hospice encourages the people on service, with the help of their families, to finish their life on their terms and to maintain a meaning or purpose in life.

In the last decade, with the growth of the hospice movement, more books are being written about the modern experience of aging and dying. These books tend to focus on the need for a transformation of medicine's role in affecting the quality of the dying experience, not just trying to prevent it. It's frustrating for any hospice staff to see how society's hesitancy to examine the experience of aging and dying has extended the suffering of terminally ill people and has denied them basic comforts that are most needed at the end of life.

I'm sure that there are several factors, but I think that the hospice movement has helped society's thinking begin to move away from the institutionalized version of aging and death. As with any change, there will be some aversion to a new way of looking at things. But those in the medical field are learning through understanding what works or does not work in our current approach to caring for those nearing the end of life. We will find better approaches to end of life care than the "Do everything" approach.

A physician I conversed with at a health fair told me that his impression of what we did was to give a patient a high dose of pain medicine and let nature take its course. Obviously, that is not true. The focus of every hospice is to respect a patient's priorities and honor what makes living worthwhile.

This physician also mentioned how hard, albeit almost impossible, it is to begin the difficult conversation of telling a person, especially one he's known for a long time, that there is no cure for their condition. He said that if not the patient, then a close family member will sometimes plead that the physician at least try to do something, anything.

The most important aspect for the physician to convey is that he is on the patient's side. Then ask the patient about specific fears and what trade-offs they are willing to make. This allows everyone involved to decide what choices would be best.

Not all end-of-life situations are hospice appropriate and it's very important to look at all sides when faced with the biggest crisis life can offer. But if it gets to the point that enough is enough, you might consider calling a hospice. The student nurse, mentioned at the beginning of this piece, learned through experience that hospice care is good care. It may be a good choice during the last stage of life.

~ I C U or the Kitchen? ~

WHERE WOULD YOU like to spend the last stage of life? My guess is that being hooked up to a bunch of machines, tubes, etc., in an ICU is not one of the places that you'd want to be. And believe it or not, most people don't want to spend their last days at the beach, nor do they want to head to Vermont in the Fall. At least, that is what those who are actually in the last stage of life tell me. It seems that most people want to do something one last time, and to do it at home. Home is where they are comfortable and that is where the memories are.

Hospice allows the patient to decide where they want to live. If they still own a home, most patients want to continue living at home. It doesn't stop there. Since it is the patient's home, if they need a hospital bed we will set it up wherever they darn well want. As a patient contact volunteer, I've visited patients whose beds were set up in the living room, unfinished basement, workshop, garage with a street rod, camper, and my favorite location, the kitchen. A patient bed in the kitchen?! Why not? That was where the action was in the patient's house and, as she told me, "I ain't dead yet."

Hospice isn't as much a medical organization focusing on an illness as it is a compassionate organization focusing on a person and their family. And nothing says family like the kitchen.

~ It's the Little Things ~

THE PATIENT WAS sitting in a wicker chair on the front porch of my hospice's facility, The Pickering House, crocheting. The patient, whom I'll call "Molly," was waiting to meet the volunteer recently assigned to her.

After the brief introduction, a few minutes of awkward silence ensued. The volunteer asked if she could bring her anything, Molly kept crocheting and said a polite, "No." The volunteer relates that, "I then shared how we sometimes bring patients pizza, fast food, or some other favorite treat if they wanted something. More silence followed. Then, in her quiet voice, she said, 'I like the iced cherry donuts from Donut World.' She seemed almost embarrassed to share this."

"I suspected that this was one of the few times she was placing her own desire first. A little while later, she went inside The Pickering House and I went to Donut World. I returned with two donuts in a bag. I walked into her room and offered them to her. She ate one donut and then said, 'I'm sorry I don't have any money with me.' I reminded her that bringing favorite treats to folks was what we did at hospice. She smiled and now seemed content accepting the gift. Without any further hesitation, she reached into the bag, pulled out the second donut and happily ate it."

The plan of care for every hospice patient where I volunteer begins with the question, "What does the patient want?" It may be as simple as a volunteer bringing two iced cherry donuts from Donut World.

~ LONELY PATIENT ~

A HOSPICE VOLUNTEER ACCEPTED an assignment to work with a person living in a nursing home. On her first visit, the volunteer announced her arrival to the employee at the nurse's station but was cautioned that there was no use visiting this particular patient because, for years, she has been uncommunicative. Heeding the advice during the initial visit, the volunteer didn't talk much. She'd occasionally asked the patient if she would like a glass of water, a story read, or anything. No reply.

The patient's bed was on the inward side of the room and the privacy curtain that divided the room was drawn around the bed. Even though it was a sunny day, her corner of the room was dim, depressing. She lay in bed, motionless, facing the wall. Watching the woman, alone in her tiny world bothered the volunteer. On the second visit, the hospice volunteer had an idea, "Would you like to look out the window?" There was a soft, "Yes."

The curtain was opened so the patient could look out the window. The patient's eyes widened and started to water. She gazed out the window seemingly in deep thought. Upon leaving, the volunteer stopped by the nurse's station to ask if the patient could be moved to a room that had a window-side bed. Eventually she was moved to such a room. To everyone's amazement the patient started to talk, albeit in short sentences.

Isn't it amazing how just spending some time with someone can literally brighten their day?

~ Massage Therapy ~

THE HOSPICE MASSAGE therapist arrived at the patient's house in order to give him his first massage. The patient needed a cane to walk and often had to keep his hand on the wall for balance. Karen, the therapist, hoped to improve the range of motion in the patient's hips and possibly improve his ability to walk. Meeting the patient, Karen was taken aback by how much he looked like the actor, Jimmy Stewart.

Karen says that with hospice patients, she takes as much or as little time as seems appropriate. There is no specified length of time for a session. In this case, Karen took more time with him since he responded to her touch. She wanted him to receive as much improvement as his health would allow.

Karen said that when she was done, the man slowly got off the table and then walked around the room, twirling his cane around his finger. He had not moved like that in a long time. What a joy it was for her to see such a positive response to her work. As the man was walking across the room, the elation he felt caused him to spontaneously start doing a little "swivel-hip" move like Elvis Presley doing the Twist. With a twinkle in his eye, he winked at his wife and said that he hadn't felt like this in years.

Karen is a perfect example of the value in taking the time needed to help a patient get some of that "zing" back in his swing and to celebrate life.

~ A LOT OF GOOD PEOPLE ~

HOW CAN ANYONE work in a hospice? I think one of the reasons is that hospice workers are in a position to help people in ways that are unique. The truth is, hospice is not as much for someone actively dying nearly as much as it is for someone who is entering the last stage of life. The last stage of life, according to Medicare, is six months. This is an estimate based on the primary doctor's belief that if the primary illness is allowed to follow its normal course the patient has six months, or less, of life remaining. For hospice, the key phrase is, "…of life remaining." Crazy as it sounds, we who are involved with hospice are all about life. And we're not kidding, because the longer someone is on service the more we can help.

When someone is fortunate enough to decide to accept hospice service before they are actively dying, we are given the opportunity to help them live. For some people, their version of living may be that they just want to go home and lead a quiet life. While some may want to visit friends, or go places they've been "meaning to visit," others may have a purpose, a goal in life that needs to be completed. Through all these situations, we are there to help.

For one of the people I accepted as a hospice volunteer, I was able to help a patient with a goal he needed to complete before he died. Through this experience, I witnessed how hospice understands the importance of living one's life and that there is still purpose to the end. As unimportant as it may seem to others the drive to complete a purpose, or goal, may be paramount to the person in their last stage of life. As what happens many times when a person on service has a goal to accomplish, my patient lived much longer than expected.

In this case, the person I accepted was a man in his 60's. At the time of his admission the patient, "Grandpa John," was alert, oriented and loved to talk. The volunteer's conversations with John covered many subjects because this man had led a full life. He was a Navy veteran, he was highly educated and he was very creative.

John also happened to be an accomplished woodworker. He'd made doll houses, bookshelves and toy chests for his children and until recently, for his grandchildren as well. As a military man, he was mission-driven. "Git 'er done" wasn't a slogan for him – it was a way of life.

On my first visit, I learned that John was on his final mission. It was a mission that would eventually take a few good men to help complete. Please pardon the generalization, but men tend to be task-oriented and relate to the importance of getting the job done, no matter what. In this case, the mission was not a dollhouse or toy chest, but a train layout. Grandpa John had made gifts for all his other grandchildren, and now his mission was to build an HO scale train layout for his youngest grandchild, a little six-year-old boy. John knew that it would be his last accomplishment on Earth and wanted it to be his own handy work.

During each weekly visit, we'd talk and he worked on the layout. He didn't want any help. After about a month or so I noticed a decline in John's health. He was now bedbound. In order to get the job done, John had his son make a small workbench to fit over the bed. At one point, John wrapped Velcro on both his wrists and the work bench so that he could control his tremulous hands. That worked well and he had made great progress but Grandpa John was gradually getting too weak to continue. His illness was taking all his energy.

It was becoming obvious that John would not be able to get his project completed. Something had to be done. I talked to John's son who convinced his dad to accept help. John's pride was put aside.

With very little model train experience but a strong desire to help, I swung into action. Knowing that a lot of help was needed, I contacted the manager of a local hobby shop who gave me the name of a local model railroad club's president. After several voice mails and a little convincing, the club president put me in touch with a club member who builds model train layouts as a sideline business. Hearing of my predicament , the man solicited the help of other club members and agreed to complete the layout quickly and at no charge! Elated, I told John the good news; the layout would be completed. Upon hearing the news, John smiled, laid his head back on his pillow and went into a peaceful sleep.

That evening visit in which Grandpa John learned that his layout would soon be complete turned out to be the last time I would see him. John passed four days later on a Saturday morning. Several weeks later the layout was finished by the model train club members who presented it to John's son. The son set it up in Grandpa's work shop and told *his* son that it was from Grandpa. And it was, both physically and spiritually.

When you understand the hospice philosophy on life, you understand that this story had a happy ending. John still had a specific goal in his life and was allowed to stay focused on it even in the last stage of his life. And against his nature, he allowed a volunteer to help him accomplish that goal. And strangers, some of whom were not enthused with end-of-life situations, rose to the occasion to assist. It reminds me of what Mr. Rogers' mom said to him when he saw disasters on the evening news. "Look at all of the good people who are helping."

There are a lot of good people in hospice, both volunteers and staff, who are helping. We understand that life has purpose and are willing to help. Especially during the last stage.

~ THE FINAL VOW ~

JUNE IS THE month for weddings and a part of weddings are the heartfelt vows. In the hospice field, we get to know the person on service and their family very well. Sometimes we are blessed to see the wedding vows fulfilled. On one consecrated evening, the hospice staff was able to witness the final vow in its most elemental form.

The wife was in my hospice facility, The Pickering House, for end-of-life care. During her stay, her hospice nurse had noticed that the patient's husband of over 50 years never left her bedside. On this particular evening, when the nurse entered the patient's room, experience told her that their final wedding vow, "...'til death do us part," was about to be fulfilled.

Seeing the unflinching devotion of the husband, the nurse knew exactly what had to be done. With the help of Pickering House aides and housekeeping staff they helped the husband get into bed to lay with his actively dying wife. Although she had not responded to any stimuli, as he lay down with her and wrapped his arms around her, her facial expression relaxed, her body relaxed, and her breathing relaxed. He held her so close that she knew she was in his arms.

No medication could ever bring that kind of comfort and peace. It was so beautiful and so heart wrenching at the same time. During this entire event, no words were spoken. The silence said everything.

Hospice understands that the end of life is a sacred experience; it's not a medical event.

~ From Music to Spirituality ~

I N ONE WAY or another we are all affected by music. Music has the power to calm a person when they are in a crisis. Any person who works in a crisis-filled occupation understands that music just seems to give what is needed at the moment.

On a late autumn afternoon, a woman came to my hospice's facility, The Pickering House, to visit her mother. The daughter was a musician so she brought her flute to play for her mom. As she played, the normally quiet environment of The Pickering House was immersed with the peaceful sound of the flute.

In Room 2, across the hall from the flutist, a distressed family was sitting at the bedside of their father. Indications were that he was in his final Hour. The man had been restless but he, as everyone else, was calmed by the music.

When she began to play "*Danny Boy*" there seemed to be a transition from music to spirituality. The shadows of late afternoon coupled with the emotion of the song created a surrealistic, yes, a heavenly ambiance.

When "*Danny Boy*" was over, there was silence. Then a voice from Room 2 said, "He's gone." For a few minutes, The Pickering House stood still. It was an intensely spiritual, beautiful stillness. The family of the deceased man believed that the flutist was an angel sent by God. No one who was there believes otherwise.

Music is a unifier because it allows all of us to experience the same emotions. At my hospice facility, musicians are always encouraged to drop in and play for a little while. You never know, someone may be restless.

~ One Last Fair Cookie ~

THE FAMILY HAD all come home to the place where they grew up. But this wasn't a particularly happy occasion, for they gathered around their mom's bed to say their good-byes. It was a beautiful Fall afternoon – clear, bright, maybe in the low 60's. "Perfect Fair weather" said one of the patient's daughters.

"Fair-time" was repeated almost in a whisper by several of those in attendance. The ensuing lively conversation began with, "Remember the time we were at the fair and…" The hospice social worker who was present felt certain that the patient was able to hear, and enjoy, the many family memories of the county fair.

One memory that kept coming up was Mom's cookies being entered in the fair every year. There was laughter while those in the room reminisced about sneaking one of her freshly baked cookies and fond memories of the aroma that wafted through the house during the last few days before the fair.

Eventually the laughter and conversation quieted down and Mom, lying in her bed, again became the focus. A change in the patient's breathing pattern told the family the Hour that everyone dreaded had come.

A granddaughter who was there had fond memories of baking cookies during those early October afternoons with her Grandma. She had her iPod with her and used her computer skills, inherent with children, and got to work making her Grandma a "virtual cookie" on her iPod. When it was done she gently placed the iPod in her Grandma's hand. The smiles soon turned to tears as she took one last breath and died. It was evident to all present that Grandma wanted one last county fair cookie. Ah, fair time.

~ Pepper ~

A S A PATIENT care volunteer, I accepted an assignment to a family who lived in the country. As anyone who lives in the country will tell you, stray animals occasionally show up on the property. In this case, a stray, shorthaired dog showed up one afternoon. They named her "Pepper" because she had a white coat with a "zillion" tiny black spots. She almost looked gray.

Pepper was afraid of everyone, especially the man of the house. Speculation was that where she grew up, the man of the house had been abusive towards her. Eventually, the man in Pepper's new family was able to gain her confidence and they became close.

Several years later the man became terminally ill and signed on to hospice service. He was lucky in that he signed on early in his last stage of life and was on our service for an extended period.

In September, when I arrived for my initial visit, Pepper was frightened of me, as puppyhood fears came rushing back. She stayed quite a distance out in the yard when I got out of my car. Experience taught me to always keep doggy treats in my car in case there were pets in the household. I placed a few "Beggin' Strips" near my car and went in. Sure enough, when I returned later the treats were gone.

For the next several months the routine gradually changed from leaving the treats near the car, to Pepper approaching the car, to eventually taking the treats out of my hand. By winter, when I arrived, Pepper would take her Beggin' Strip and wait near the front door to be let in with me. At a comfortable distance, however.

She would lie in the patient's room while I was there, but she never got physically close enough to be petted. By June, the man's health deteriorated to the point that the hospice nurse knew it wouldn't be long. Pepper also knew. She seemed to look to me for help. Dogs sense when life is ending and as her owner's health worsened, Pepper would meet me as I parked my car, then walk in to the house with me. She would lie next to me at the patient's bedside.

Three months after the man's death I came by to make my first bereavement visit with the widow. While we were talking at the kitchen table, Pepper came in and laid her head across my feet. She didn't budge. It was as if she needed to hear what was being discussed.

Most dogs, and I guess maybe a few cats, grieve when they lose their owner. Some dogs don't seem to show any reaction, some show a few behavior changes and some, like the one lying on my feet, grieve a lot. Possibly it's the degree of closeness in the relationship between pet and patient that determines the level of grief. Pepper, lying at my feet, needed to be included during my bereavement visit.

~ Respite ~

ONE OF THE primary functions of a stand-alone hospice facility is that it offers respite to caregivers by affording the patient a five day stay, depending upon the particular hospice' protocol. That's nice, but what is "respite"? (Pronounced *ress pit*). Other words for respite are: breather, pause, recess, rest, and time out. Most people, when they come to grips with their situation, prefer to spend their last days at home. By the time they get to this stage of life, they are tired of going somewhere into a medical facility to be treated and tired of the recuperation time after the treatment. They just want to be comfortable in familiar surroundings.

Allowing someone to spend their life in familiar surroundings is exactly what most hospices do. We encourage the patient to stay where they'd like to stay. When the choice is to stay in their home, or maybe a family member's home, then those family members will become involved in the patient's care. Hospice personnel will show the family members how to do as much as they want to do for the patient. But since it often becomes a 24-hour-a-day proposition they become tired, both emotionally and physically. When that time comes, the hospice will bring the patient to a palliative care area of a hospital or nursing home. Some hospices, such as mine, will bring the patient to their own hospice house so that the caregivers can get some respite, or a break, from the stress of patient care.

During what is normally a five-day respite stay, hospice staff will give the patient more attention and better care than they ever thought possible. And that in itself is respite for the family.

~ Security Prayer ~

EVERYONE WANTS A feeling of security. As a serious illness progresses, it can be especially hard on men as their ability to drive, to fix things, etc. slowly diminishes. I think that not being able to use the remote is one of the last abilities to go.

Talking to a patient a few years ago, he mentioned how nice everything in his house was set up by the hospice staff. The hospital bed in the home, the medicine set up by day and dosage, the schedules of nurse visits written down, all helped to keep things in order. Interestingly, he told me, "You know, this hospital bed seems to make it easier to sleep. Seems weird, but when the side rails are raised, they give me a nice feeling of security."

I happened to read an article on prayer by John V. Chervokas and in it was a prayer that dealt with the same issue. It reads:

"I trust it's not a reversion to my crib days, God, but I must confess it feels so good to have the sides of my bed pulled up at night. I gaze at the bars and, as my eyes grow heavy rather than feeling any cooped-up sensation, I rest safe and secure and warm. With You involved in every phase of my life I'll strive to remember I need never be fearful. I'll try not to forget that in Your loving care 'the sides' are always up. Amen."

According to that patient, hospice offers peace and security when it is needed most.

~ Subtle Spirituality ~

I AM OFTEN asked if I've ever experienced anything "spiritual" or "supernatural" while volunteering at my local hospice. Yes, I have. And I know all our staff who work directly with patients and families have, as well. Usually it happens the same way that God works in all of us; by slowly, inconspicuously putting us in a position to do His work. It's up to us to be alert and to respond.

One occurrence that I will always remember happened on one of the first warm days of Spring. Being in the construction industry at the time, warm weather meant business. I was busy that day. I was also a hospice patient care volunteer and was assigned to a man in his 50's. My normal schedule was to visit him every Tuesday evening.

Since I had been associated with him for the six months he'd been on service, we became good friends. The hospice office called me and said that my patient, "Denny," had started the dying process. His family was gathering. His wife said that he was asking for me.

I left work early and went straight to the nursing home where he had been living for the past week. Before that, he was living in a fairly dark, cluttered sleeping room on the second floor of a rundown duplex. My purpose as a volunteer was to stay with him so his wife could go out for a while. He was a veteran of Vietnam and was one of the war veterans who just couldn't leave the war behind. His life had been one of turmoil sprinkled liberally with alcohol.

When I arrived, a group of about 10 people were on the front porch of the nursing home. Those on the porch were Denny's wife, brothers, an aunt and a few others who had come over to say their good-byes. Since they were outside, I thought that maybe my patient had died before I got there. Nope. They had ordered pizza and the driver was evidently running a little late.

The transition from the bright, sunny weather and the almost party-like atmosphere on the front porch to the sacred radiance of his room was almost too much to comprehend. Only those fortunate enough to have been in a room when someone is dying understand the feeling of being there. The room was spotless, and everything was either white or pastel green. Denny was shaven, his hair was combed and he was in a clean hospital-type gown. I hate to say it, but I initially didn't recognize him. During the time that I knew him he always had a scruffy two or three-day beard, shoulder length hair, and generally wouldn't allow hospice aides to bathe him.

What immediately caught my eye was his water glass sitting on the bedside table. A sunbeam was shining on that glass like a spotlight on a singer at center stage. As I reverently entered his room he slowly turned his head towards me. His eyes were wide and his mouth was open. In the last hours of life, there is rarely enough energy left to talk, but I sensed that he was afraid to die. I talked to him for a few minutes, pushed his hair back a little bit and patted his hand. I tried to reassure him that everything was, going to be okay, that soon he would be in the arms of his Savior.

His eyes went down then slowly found mine. I remembered that at one-time Denny had told me that he never went to church and that he was "too much of a sinner." He doubted that he was going to Heaven. Now, thinking of that conversation, I told Denny about what Jesus said to the two criminals as the three of them were being crucified. The one on His left rejected Jesus, even in his last hour, while the one on His right humbly asked, "Jesus, remember me when You come into your Kingdom." Jesus answered him by saying, "I tell you the truth, today you will be with Me in Paradise." (Luke 23:42-43)

My patient maintained his wide-eyed stare at me. He needed assurance. He needed to know that he would be going to Heaven. I told him that his emptiness and fear were a perfect match for the abundance and love of Jesus. I assured him that everything would be okay.

The beam of light streaming in from the window illuminating the water glass on the bedside table was now the only thing that I saw in the room. An overwhelming urge directed me to reach over his bed and dip my fingers in the water. I told if he felt ready I was going to baptize him. He looked towards the ceiling, then closed his eyes. Touching his head, heart, and each shoulder I whispered, "I baptize you in the name of the Father, the Son, and the Holy Spirit." The outside corner of his left eye looked moist, although in the last hours of life the body is too dehydrated for tears. I rationalized that I used too much water. He kept his eyes closed, so I touched his forearm and left.

Out on the front porch the pizza had arrived. His wife thanked me for stopping by and asked me how Denny was doing. I told her, "He is at peace." It was 6 p.m. The hospice office called me later that evening and said that Denny had died at 6:45. He died about 45 minutes after his baptism.

A few minutes after that call, it dawned on me that at least ten people had arrived to be with Denny on his last day on earth. Yet, no one was in the room except for me when he needed to prepare to enter the Kingdom. How would the pizza delivery person know that by arriving later than expected, he was a part of God's plan to help someone into Heaven?

Before I came into the subtle spirituality of hospice work I might not have baptized Denny. I had briefly thought to myself, "What if I'm not allowed, or authorized, to baptize someone? I haven't been to seminary, I have no training." However, in this case I just knew that it had to be done.

The hospice where I volunteer is not a religious organization but in the waning moments of life, spiritual comfort is at the heart of what we do.

~ Someone Understands ~

I LOVE THE county fair. And it's not just the food that I like about it. Don't get me wrong, one of the main reasons I like the fair is definitely the food. But I also really enjoy talking with everyone there. The hospice where I volunteer sets up a display in the Art Hall every year. Every year I spend as much time as I can at our display because of the people who stop by to talk.

Anyone who walks by and has had no experience with hospice will take one of our pens, a post-it notepad, and maybe a hand sanitizer. However, the people who have had an experience with hospice, either through a family member or acquaintance, usually have something to say. And it's always nice. Every so often, someone will have a question about what we do.

One of our volunteers was at our booth one evening and a woman came up to say thanks for our care of her mother. What got the volunteer's attention was the woman said that suddenly there was someone who understood exactly what we were facing. That, to me, is the hallmark of hospice care; we understand what you are facing. We don't focus on the illness, we focus on you.

Caring for a family member with a serious illness can cause tremendous stress. The comedian Jeff Foxworthy said that you know you are a caregiver if you start dividing your M&M's into a pill box. Before something like that happens call hospice. Suddenly someone will understand.

~ The Air Mattress ~

L IFE CAN HAVE funny moments, even in its last stage. A middle-aged man, to whom I was assigned as a patient-contact volunteer, was living at home. His bed was equipped with an air mattress that had a small electric air compressor plugged into the wall. The compressor would allow the patient to control the firmness of the mattress. During my evening visit, a severe thunderstorm came through and knocked out the power. The lights went out and his compressor stopped. In the darkness, I could barely hear a muffled, "Help me, I'm over here."

I turned my flash light (part of my emergency kit) towards his voice and all that was visible were his hands and feet protruding from the middle crease of the mattress. Basically, he sank to the bottom and the mattress pad folded up around him. He was in no danger of suffocating because there was not enough material to cover his face.

There was a manual foot pedal that I pumped to quickly inflate the mattress back to its correct size. As luck would have it, his grown daughter arrived back home but just that time. Seeing me stomping on the foot pedal and her Dad slightly bouncing to the rhythm of the air entering the air mattress, she burst out laughing. She thought we were having some sort of hoedown. Once the bed was inflated, he joined his daughter in laughing. Neither could stop. He said, "That was the most fun I've had in years. Let's do it again!" It was initially a scary situation, but my patient, as patients often do, taught me to handle life as it comes and enjoy what happens. He showed me that sometimes things that seem scary often are not.

~ THE FINAL ACT OF LOVE ~

W HEN THE DYING process starts naturally, it cannot be stopped. We can try to alter or interfere with the process but it cannot be stopped. When it starts, the loving thing to do is give comfort.

When a person enters the final stage of life, the dying process begins. During this stage of life two different dynamics are at work. On the physical plane, the body begins the final process of shutting down, which will end when all the physical systems cease to function. Usually this is an orderly and undramatic progressive series of physical changes which are not medical emergencies requiring invasive interventions. These physical changes are a normal, natural way in which the body prepares itself to stop and the most appropriate kinds of responses are comfort-enhancing measures.

The other dynamic of the dying process is at work on the emotional-spiritual-mental plane, and is a different kind of process. The "spirit" of the dying person begins the final process of release from the body, its immediate environment, and all attachments. This release also tends to follow its own priorities, which may include the resolution of whatever is unfinished of a particular nature and reception of permission to "let go" from family members. The most appropriate kinds of responses to the emotional-spiritual-mental changes are those which support and encourage this release and transition.

The experience we call death occurs when the body completes its natural process of shutting down, and when the spirit completes its natural process of reconciling and finishing. Your local hospice shows you different techniques to use in order to comfort your loved one through this process. Comforting your loved one during this time is the final act of love.

~ Yes, The Little Things ~

ONE OF THE reasons that hospice impresses people with its level of care is that we, as hospice people, understand the last stage of life. I mean really understand it. The truth is that when confronted with a terminal diagnosis, everyone at some point must accept that life does have an end. Hospice understands that what seem to be the littlest things to us may, in fact, be of utmost importance to someone who is terminally ill.

Years ago, we had an Air Force Korean War veteran on service. The bedridden patient mentioned that he missed seeing an F-86 jet fighter like the one he flew in that war. As his hospice patient-contact volunteer, I happened to know a nationally recognized model builder who lived in the area. I made arrangements with him, also an Air Force veteran, to bring over some of his F-86 models to show the man.

We met the patient in his home's large recreation room where he had hospice set up his bed. Upon seeing the expertly made F-86 Sabre Jet models, some featured in national magazines, the patient was ecstatic. The planes were laid out on a table and the stories began.

Their conversation was intense. There were combat stories with the patient moving his hands around describing how he attacked a Russian MiG in a dogfight. More dog fights were re-enacted, there was laughter, chatter and there was silence as tears were held back. I'm sure that if I had quietly gone home and come back two hours later, the modeler and veteran wouldn't have known it.

Months later the veteran's grateful widow was amazed that somehow we knew how important it was for her husband to see an F-86. Hospice knows that, yes, the little things are important.

~ Why Won't They Eat ~

PART OF MY duties at the hospice where I volunteer is to talk to every civic and church group and every type of club in the community about the goodness of hospice care. When I begin my talk I usually begin by asking if anyone has questions about hospice. I know that sounds backwards but it's the only way for me to find out what they want to know regarding hospice (if anything) and what are their misconceptions about hospice. If I may generalize, anyone who has not witnessed hospice compassion first hand will have misgivings about it, if not misconceptions.

At one presentation, a man said that he felt guilty because while he was caring for his ailing mother she came to the point where she wouldn't eat. She had been ill for quite some time and eventually became bedridden. As she continued to decline in health, he had to feed her. It wasn't that long before she refused to eat at all. His effort to feed her was repeated at mealtime for several days. According to him, she died within a week or so. He felt that because he couldn't get her to eat he had in effect starved her.

Eating at the end of life is not a subject that I discuss too often at a presentation but, because of his statement and his continuing guilt from his feeling that he had caused his mother to die, I talked about it. The truth is, there are many normal activities that we have done all our life that are no longer relevant at the end of life, and that may be the root of many hospice misconceptions.

A hospice patient differs from a healthy person, or even someone who is very sick because, depending upon their progress in the last stage of life their body may be in the process of shutting down. In the last stage of life, the body knows that it's dying. Since food is necessary to sustain life, the body knows that food is no longer necessary and, therefore, rejects it. There is no more need for nutrition. The sensation of not wanting food is very similar to when you have an upset stomach and you are not interested in eating.

During your last stage of life, you are a different person. This is especially so with your physical qualities; your metabolism is different, your bodily functions are different, and your organs may begin the process of turning off. The same type of medical attention that you received through your life up to this point doesn't work anymore.

The hospice where I volunteer gives an information packet to the ill person and their family containing a sheet that details why food and liquids should be restricted or removed from a patient's intake. This packet is a good example of one of the hallmarks of hospice compassion; we give the family instructions on how to care for the loved one (if they want the information) and, most importantly, why certain things should or shouldn't be done. The following few paragraphs contain information taken from that new-patient packet.

Sometimes your loved one will not want to eat and drink due to the body slowing down with fewer physical needs. The person does not need calories to convert to energy anymore. As death approaches, dehydration occurs naturally from not enough food or liquid intake. Occasional thirst, dry mouth, and changes in mental status sometimes happen. The mental changes, while upsetting to you, bring relief to your loved one by lessening their awareness of suffering.

The administration of IV fluids may produce a feeling of well-being, but it's usually a fleeting sensation. In time, artificial hydration is likely to heighten the discomfort of a terminally ill patient and often increases underlying symptoms. Reducing fluid intake decreases lung congestion and coughs.

Unless kidney function has declined, IV fluids increase urine output, often creating a need for an indwelling catheter. Fluid deprivation eliminates the frequent use of a urinal or bedpan and the discomfort that goes along with it. IVs can contribute to increased chances of developing pressure sores, and swelling. They can also cause increased pressure on tumors, organs, and nerves, causing increased pain. Dehydration diminishes the risk.

Mouth discomfort, then, is dehydration's only drawback. Good mouth care and comfort measures bring relief. To ease a patient's mouth discomfort, use moisturizers and frequent rinses with nonalcoholic mouthwashes. You may also offer ice chips and the patient's favorite liquid frequently. Apply lip balm or petroleum jelly to chapped, dry lips but avoid lemon and glycerin swabs because they promote dryness. Accompanied by comfort measures and emotional support, dehydration is a humane therapeutic response to terminal illness.

We all know the old saying that there are no absolutes in life except death, and taxes. So, to backtrack just a bit, depending upon the patient's progress in the last stage of life, there are foods and fluids that can be given to a patient that will give them comfort. When relevant, adequate nutrition while on hospice care is important. The patient will let you know when enough is enough. It is extremely hard on those close to the patient to restrict intake, but your loved one knows when their Hour is approaching.

Offer foods, or snacks that are a favorite of the patient. Sometimes cold foods such as ice cream or a fruit-flavored slushy may help. Try offering frequent, small meals and maybe take a break while eating. Hard candy or chewing gum may help to keep the mouth moist as will rinsing the mouth frequently.

So much of what hospice suggests for a patient may not seem logical at first, especially when it comes to eating. However, a person in the last stage of life is different, both physically and emotionally, than when they were healthy. It is important to know that everything hospice does for a patient and their family is driven by our desire to comfort everyone involved. We will help you.

~ I'll Wear This One ~

A S SHE STOOD there waiting for the ceremony to begin, Kristen was calming herself down. This was her Big Day, her wedding day. Helen, or "Nanny" as everyone knew her, had been waiting for this day and she wasn't going to miss this moment for the world. Her only grandchild, Zach, was the groom and her sole wish in life had been to watch him get married. Nanny was brought right up front so that she wouldn't miss a thing. Zach gingerly pinned a corsage on "his Nan." Nanny's only child, Christina, and Christina's husband, George, made themselves comfortable next to her.

The pastor was ready. Kristen's Dad, Mark, was ready to walk her down the "aisle." The wedding party was ready. Now all they had to do was wait until Nanny was ready. Her illness had been making her very tired. Just past 9:30, she stirred a bit and it looked like as good a time as any to begin the ceremony.

This wedding was a profoundly spiritual event. In order to make it happen, every participant including the couple, their family, and friends, and even a few people who didn't know the couple demonstrated selfless, sacrificial, and unconditional love. The serenity of Agape love filled the room. In every marriage ceremony, there is the public declaration of the couple's true love for each other. But at some point in every marriage, when problems are encountered, sometimes the vows hold true and sometimes they don't. Truth is you never know if it's true love until things go wrong. In Kristen and Zach's case, things did go horribly wrong, a mere 36 hours before the ceremony.

This wedding had been "in the works" for over four months. It was planned for New Year's Eve. Yet now the marriage ceremony was taking place at 9:30 in the morning on the Tuesday after Easter, nine months early. As recently as the previous Thursday, Holy Thursday,

Kristen had big plans to spend the day with Nanny shopping for bridesmaid dresses. But Nanny cancelled saying she was just too tired. Nanny too tired?! Something was wrong. Nanny had never been too tired to help anyone, let alone anyone who wanted to go shopping for bridesmaid dresses.

On Good Friday, Nanny stayed home and rested. Zach grew concerned. On Holy Saturday morning Zach took her to Urgent Care. Tests showed that she had a very high white blood cell count. Alarmed, a few phone calls were made and she was sent up to "The James," the highly-esteemed cancer research hospital on the campus of the Ohio State University. She was admitted.

On Easter Sunday morning, the diagnosis was determined; Nanny had a rare, aggressive form of cancer. Nanny? Please, God, no. Not her. The doctors tried to be positive, but could only promise maybe two weeks of life for her. Numbed by what they had just heard, the family gathered around Nanny. Searching for words, they gave her the prognosis. Her immediate reply was, "Oh, I'll miss the wedding." Hearing what Nanny said gave Kristen a jolt. "Nanny's only concern was our wedding." She felt empty.

Kristen, Zach, and Christina were now faced with difficult decisions. What treatments were available? Would she be able to tolerate them? Would she have to move into a nursing home? Kristen knew that she would have to put her wedding plans on hold to help care for Nanny. In this moment of crisis, they forgot that Nanny was still Nanny. She would make the decision for them. She said all her life she had seen many of her stricken friends spend the rest of their life trying not to die rather than trying to enjoy the time that was remaining. So, she was adamant; no chemo and no treatments of any sort. "Please, just call FairHoPe Hospice." It was unsettling at first but if that was what Nanny wanted, then that was what she would get. Now the course was clear: get Nanny to FairHoPe's in patient facility, The Pickering House, and try to make her as comfortable as possible.

The FairHoPe social worker arrived at "The James" on Easter afternoon to admit her. Once the social worker heard about the situation, she sensed how important the wedding was to Nanny.

And experience told her that Nanny was very close to the end of her life. She suggested that possibly the wedding should be moved up to the next day or two. "We'll help." she added.

The family was caught off guard; have the wedding in a few days?! And hospice will help? Kristen and Zach looked at each other. It was up to Kristen. Knowing all that Nanny had given to others without a thought about herself, the decision was quick. "Certainly we can give her our wedding. Let's do it." The doctors at The James were enthusiastic about the idea. Nanny was scheduled to arrive at The Pickering House on Monday and the wedding was now scheduled for Tuesday.

Once the decision was made to have the wedding, things began to happen. With less than two days before the wedding, a short list of who to invite was drawn up and phoned invitations were made. When asked what time the wedding would be, all anyone could tell them was, "In the morning." Nanny's health was continuing to deteriorate by the hour and no one knew what to expect on Tuesday morning. Since no one knew exactly when the marriage vows would be exchanged, no one knew when the Reception would begin. Or if there would be one.

On the Monday morning before a Tuesday wedding, there isn't a lot of time to get things done. But as it turned out, this event had all the makings of a somewhat traditional, albeit frantic, wedding. Deanna, Kristen's mom, let her borrow a pearl necklace. Well, something borrowed will help. A family friend donated the handkerchief she used years ago to hold her wedding bouquet so that Kristen would have something for her bouquet. That is, should they be able to find any flowers in the morning. That made something old for the wedding. (Do you see a pattern developing?)

"What do we need? What do we need?" was a question often asked that afternoon. "The ring!" Deanna went to Kohl's to see what she could find. Since there was no time to shop around she ended up buying the only wedding band that was in Kristen's size. Ah, something new. For the wedding dress, Zach suggested, "I like this one." It was her floral print dress with blue flowers that she'd worn on several dates.... something blue.

Kristen and Zach were at the Courthouse at 8 on the dot Monday morning in order to get the marriage license. Then to the florist who happened to have some pink and white carnations. They were arranged into a bridal bouquet in record time. Everyone involved did whatever was needed. The Pickering House staff pitched in to move furniture and help make everything just perfect. In fact, the FairHoPe Hospice nurse even adjusted the time that Nanny's medications would be administered so that she would be at her highest level of alertness during the morning.

With CD music playing, the hospice staff wheeled Nanny's bed into the Sun Room of the Pickering House. When the ceremony began, Nanny was prone in her bed. But when she heard the couple begin to exchange vows, she sat up and was very aware of what was going on. Her daughter, Christina, was at her bedside assisting her. She made it!

The Reception became an open house type of affair with more friends coming in as more found out about what was going on. Nanny remained at the Reception for a bit, then was taken back to her room. Out of respect, only a few people at a time would go to Nanny's room.

By evening the lights in the Sun Room of The Pickering House where the wedding took place, were dimmed. Everyone had gone home and Nanny was peacefully sleeping. The FairHoPe staff made accommodations so that Christina could stay at her mom's bedside and Kristen and Zach could sleep in the room, as well. In the stillness of 2:00 the next morning, the nurse gently woke them. "She's gone…"

There were tears, prayers, and there was silence. And you know what? Nanny was still Nanny. Even in dying she was giving of herself. She waited to die until April 8th so that April 7th would be Zach and Kristen's Anniversary exclusively, not the anniversary that would always be remembered with "…and Nanny died that day, too." FairHoPe's staff has seen too many patients speed up or slow down their own dying process to think otherwise.

Kristen still wears the (fairly inexpensive) wedding band that her mom bought at Kohl's knowing that Zach will buy her an expensive, real wedding band for one of their anniversaries. But Kristen said until then she'll continue to wear the one she has because, "This one is priceless."

~ ALL OF THIS IS FOR YOU ~

"**T**HIS WHOLE ROOM is mine?!" exclaimed the new patient as she entered her room in the temporary stay hospice home. She was clearly amazed at the size of the room where she was going to be living for the next few days. There was plenty of room for family and friends to gather. "Yes, all this is just for you," her hospice social worker told her.

The hospice where I volunteer has a temporary stay hospice home. All twelve of the home's patient rooms are single occupancy, so when a person stays there for a few days, the whole room is theirs. But more than that, even if someone on hospice service never spends any time there, hospice still gives them the room they need to live comfortably. Should the ill person remain in their home, hospice will set up the hospital bed (if needed) in any room of the house that is desired.

Until a family has experienced hospice care, you just don't realize how much "room" you will be given. Most importantly, room will be given so that you can gather as a family again. Hospice will give you room to take care of your loved one to the degree that you feel comfortable. Your nurse or aide will show you as many techniques as you'd like to know in order to properly care for your loved one yourself. And hospice will give you and your family the room to talk about your spirituality if you would like to do so.

Yes, all of this is just for you. When you reach the point of exhaustion, when enough is enough, call hospice. You will get all the room that you need.

~ TIME ~

EVERY WEEK, THE hospice where I volunteer has a team meeting. The purpose of the meeting is for staff to gather and discuss the past week's patient oriented activities, new admissions, and to discuss those currently on service. During this meeting, the thank you cards received during the past week are passed around. There is always quite a stack of them. I thought it's interesting that on the surface hospice seems to do so little, medically, for people yet they receive so many thank you cards from our patients' families. The reason is one word, "time."

A hospice nurse has the time during a home visit to sit at a patient's bedside and talk about family. Hospice aides have time to bathe a patient, do their hair, and put on their favorite perfume, even though it looks like they may only have a few days of life remaining. Hospice volunteers have time to feed lunch to an ALS patient even though it may take two hours. Even when someone is only considering calling, a hospice social worker, normally the first to meet with the family, compassionately take as much time as it takes to ease the fears of the family when signing on a family member.

A hospice chaplain has time to sit, listen, cry, and laugh as a patient tells their life story. And the physicians associated with the hospice where I volunteer make house calls, when needed, and listen to the concerns of everyone in the family.

In a time of crisis, hospice has all the time you need.

~ What a Day for a Picnic ~

WHAT A DAY for a picnic! It was a wonderful warm, sunny summer afternoon. All the "fixin's" were brought to the big event in a classic picnic basket covered by a red and white checkered table cloth. You'd almost expect to see Red Riding Hood skipping along. The blanket was spread, paper plates, Styrofoam cups and plastic ware were placed. Since they didn't want to use a table, the items had to be placed carefully on the blanket so that nothing would tip over. There was a delightful "o-o-h-h-h" or an "oh, goody" as each item was taken out of the basket.

It was a basic picnic, nothing fancy. Just a simple menu of sandwiches, chips, and drinks. But it also triggered a tearful, overwhelming sense of joy in the recipient. There were tears because the picnic was a total surprise. And just how do you surprise someone with a picnic? Easy – you have it for a person on hospice service at a hospice facility... in their room.

The story began the day before during a hospice volunteer's visit with a patient at the hospice home. As the patient was reminiscing with her volunteer, Margie, she talked about how all her life she had enjoyed picnics. Sadly, now that she was ill, and bedridden, she knew that she would never go on another picnic. On her way home Margie thought, "Why not bring a picnic to the patient?" It was that simple.

Hospice celebrates life and what better way to celebrate than with a picnic?

~ Why Have Doctors on Staff? ~

I WAS TALKING to someone at a health fair and they couldn't understand why a hospice would have doctors on staff. The person's thinking was that since hospice doesn't try to cure patients, it doesn't need doctors. It's true that in its infancy, the hospice movement was perceived as anti-physician and they didn't use them. That was most likely because the first duty of a doctor has always been to focus on curing their patient and the only thing that people thought that a hospice did was let people die. However, then as now, doctors not only focus on curing but also focus on comforting their patients. It just so happens that comfort is the number one focus of hospice doctors. They are very good at it.

To dispel any misconceptions, every hospice has a physician on staff or, at least, under contract to help when needed. It's required by Medicare mandates. But that does not mean you necessarily have to give up your relationship with a trusted family doctor should you choose hospice compassion. It may come as a surprise to some, but their family doctor often has the option to maintain care of their patient when they sign on to hospice care.

It's similar to when you are seeing a specialist. The specialist tends to your serious illness while your family doctor continues to care for other maladies. More doctors are obtaining the hospice certification because hospice is recognized as a specialty of care. The hospice specialty is the last stage of life with the emphasis being the last "stage" and not just the last few days of life.

Accepting hospice is always your decision. Hospice can step in when your doctor and you decide that the best course is to stop ineffective treatment and refocus on pain management and comfort. Generally, once someone makes a referral to hospice and the family doctor concurs, the doctor will advise the hospice doctor as to the diagnosis (identity of the terminal illness) and prognosis (prediction about what the outcome will be.). The family doctor may also issue orders for medications, give patient and family information, and forward the patient's medical history and records to the hospice. The referring doctor will also certify that their patient and family understand the disease and prognosis.

In my opinion, being a family practice physician has to be a challenging career. On a day-to-day basis, the family doctor is presented with a myriad of symptoms from a variety of patients who range in age from infant to geriatric. The doctor is faced with vague descriptions from patients of symptoms requiring that the physician be perceptive as to what the real problem may be. A family doctor may also face time constraints presented by the activity in the practice's office. There always seems to be the next patient waiting.

In the case of a hospice doctor, they have as much time as a patient needs. Besides hospice doctors having time, they have another advantage in that the types of symptoms that arise due to a particular terminal illness are similar from one patient to another. Not exactly the same, but similar. A terminal illness, whether it's cancer, end stage heart disease, or any of a multitude of diseases, follows a certain pattern.

As the end of life approaches, the body turns itself off in a somewhat prescribed manner. As such, the medical profession has developed standard protocols that are effective and appropriate for the treatment of the symptoms of each terminal illness. However, within protocols, the plan of care is truly unique to the individual patient receiving the care, albeit similar to others with the same illness.

Most hospices have a willingness to discuss what everyone involved wants to do and then meet that expectation. The combination of interactions is almost limitless as to what degree of involvement the family doctor may have with the hospice doctor. The important aspect is that they both work together for the good of the patient.

The role of any doctor in hospice care is to use expertise in comfort care. The doctor involved may be the hospice's doctor, your family doctor, or a combination of both. What is most important to remember is that hospice care is care on your terms.

~ WHEN MOST NEEDED ~

WHEN SOMEONE SIGNS on to hospice compassion, part of our admitting regimen is to inquire about their current spiritual comfort level. We are interested in comforting the whole person physically, emotionally, and spiritually. If the patient has a church family we contact their clergy and offer our assistance, if needed. Sometimes the patient has no church family in which case one of our chaplains will offer their services.

Several years ago, one of my hospice's chaplains, Karl Hartmann, was asked to visit a Catholic woman who was on our service. She was unresponsive. Karl's experience told him that even though she did not respond to anyone's voice there was a good chance that she could still hear him.

Being versed in most Christian denominations Karl knew that the Catholic Faith has several common prayers said in every Catholic's prayer life. He wanted to use a prayer that the patient would be familiar with, and thus be a comfort to her. So, Karl brought a copy of the traditional Catholic prayer, the "Hail Mary," with him when he visited.

Quietly he entered her room, announced that he was there, and then pulled up a chair to sit at her bedside. He began to recite the "Hail Mary" and noticed that the patient began to silently mouth the prayer with him. Karl then began to pray the Lord's Prayer and she said it right along with him.

Karl has always said that as a chaplain his job is to comfort people where they are and as they are. By reciting a familiar prayer Karl comforted the woman when she needed it the most; during the few remaining days of her life.

~ ERNIE AND I ~

OVER A PERIOD of several months, one of my hospice's patient-contact volunteers, Pat, had made frequent trips to the nursing home to visit his patient. The patient, "Ernie," only had one living relative, a daughter who lived on the coast and hadn't visited in a long time. As is common at the end of life, Ernie slept a lot. When he was awake, he usually stared into the distance. Pat dutifully came in, sat with the man for the agreed-upon length of stay, then left. He hated to admit it, but during the last few visits he considered not visiting.

"Who does this benefit, anyway?" he'd ask himself.

Quickly feeling remorse for his thought, he knew that as a volunteer his singular purpose was to be there. Pat knew that sometimes the benefit of his efforts might not be too obvious.

As he entered one evening, the facility's nurse stopped Pat and told him Ernie's Hour was approaching. The disquieting news abruptly changed everything, i.e., should he go in and visit as planned or just go back home? As a hospice volunteer, Pat knew that he needed to be with Ernie. He softly entered the dimly lit room. The slow, rhythmic sound of the oxygen concentrator told Pat that Ernie was near the end. He reverently placed his chair at Ernie's bedside and sat down.

Uncharacteristically for anyone being at the end of life, Ernie looked straight at Pat. He closed his eyes for quite a while, then opened them and again looked at Pat. On impulse, Pat held the man's hand, leaned close to him and in a soft undertone, prayed the Lord's Prayer. Ernie whispered, "Thank you, and good-bye." Pat was stunned, Ernie hadn't spoken in weeks.

In the stillness of the nursing home late that evening Ernie died. Later, as Pat walked through the darkness to his car, his eyes reddened as he realized the answer to his question, who does this benefit, was "Ernie and I."

~ He Had Purpose ~

S EVERAL YEARS AGO, a person on my hospice's service was brought to our facility in order to give his family a break from the constant care giving. The person's terminal diagnosis was a heart condition. Fortunately, he signed on soon enough that he was still ambulatory, meaning that he could walk, and he was also alert and oriented.

During his stay, the second session of a six-session training class for new volunteers, being held at the facility, had begun. The volunteer coordinator, who facilitated the training, knew that this man who was on service had experience as a substitute teacher. Additionally, he had taught the Bible at his church. So, she decided to ask the patient if he would like to teach a class about hospice from the patient's perspective. He said that he wasn't doing anything else that night, so why not?

The patient spoke from the heart when he talked to the new volunteers about how his illness had affected him and his family. He answered questions about fear and spirituality.

The next day, when the transport ambulance came to return the patient to his home, the attendant couldn't believe it was the same person who he had dropped off five days earlier. The patient enthusiastically told the attendant that he'd been promoted to a teacher and had the certificate from the volunteer coordinator to prove it. He had purpose!

It has been said that the meaning of life is to find your gift, while the purpose of life is to give it away. Hospice allows the patient opportunity, when signed on early enough, to give his gift away. Yes, even at the end.

~ Back Into Perspective ~

FOR OUR FIRST Christmas together my wife and I decided that we couldn't afford a Christmas tree. But a few days before Christmas I noticed a small – well, very small – tree in the back of a Christmas tree lot. It was only about two feet high and the price was $1. That was cheap even then, so I bought it. My wife was elated to have our first Christmas tree.

That tree reminded me of Charlie Brown's little tree in the annual TV special, "A Charlie Brown Christmas." If you've seen the show, you'll recall that Charlie Brown becomes disillusioned with what Christmas seems to have become. He decides to buy a real Christmas tree in the hope it will bring back that feeling of the old Christmas. Like Charlie Brown's tree, ours was a puny, forlorn tree but it brought a decorous feel to what had looked like a bleak Christmas.

If you have suffered the loss of a loved one during this past year, the holidays will be different. Even if it was the loss of a job, divorce, or your health due to an illness, your life has been turned upside down. The holidays can be wonderful again but they will never be the same. Probably the most important thing to remember is that if you don't want to do anything you don't have to. There is little, if anything that you *have* to do during the holidays.

But remember that the littlest things, sometimes as simple as a little Christmas tree, can put life back into perspective. Everything will be okay.

~ THEY DO GRIEVE ~

I'VE HEARD THAT old age is defined as being 15 years older than your current age. Well, according to that definition I have fifteen years before I'm old. And speaking of being old, it seems that when someone thinks of hospice they associate us with old people. To a degree that is true since many of our patients are older.

Since a lot of our patients are older, many are grandparents. And when they die they leave behind their grandchildren. The grandchildren are often the forgotten grievers. Children may appear to be unaffected by the loss of a grandparent so we may think that they don't grieve. They do grieve. It's just that children do not grieve the same way that adults do so it may not be easily recognizable.

Young people in their teens and younger are affected by a death. They just don't have the vocabulary to explain what they are feeling, nor do they have the life experiences to understand what has happened. And sometimes in an effort to protect children from the pain of grief we may inadvertently teach children to suppress or hide their grief rather than release it.

The hospice where I work and volunteer has a grief support team dedicated to educating children and their families on how to release their tears, pain, and anger after experiencing a loss. If you have experienced a loss in your family that may have affected your children, or hear of a loss experienced by one of your children's classmates, think of hospice.

~ Graduations ~

SPRING IS THE season for graduations and graduations are a part of life. And who knows more about life than an organization that assists people at the end of theirs? Consider who would know more about marriage than someone who works in the divorce field. A divorce lawyer told me that it's normal for acquaintances to get married, but you really have to know someone to divorce them. Who would know more about the stupidity of texting and driving than the EMTs who respond to vehicle crashes that are a result of distracted driving?

Yes, we in the hospice field have a lot of experience with graduations. We have actually graduated some of our patients from our service. Say what? Hospice graduates patients?! Yes, if someone's health improves while on our service they may no longer show symptoms of approaching eminent death. When that happens, they may not be appropriate for hospice care, so we dismiss them from our service. They are just too healthy to be on service. That, in the business, is known as "graduating" off hospice.

When thinking of graduating off hospice service, one patient who immediately comes to mind lived in a nursing home. Her name was Gladys and she was 102 years old. Before she came on service Gladys was, in her own words, "...beginning to wear out." Well, as statistics from all over the country have shown, when a patient is on hospice service early enough in what is considered their last stage of life, their health tends to improve. Note that I said their health tends to improve – they are not cured. And whether their health improves or just stabilizes, all studies have shown that they live longer on hospice service than their doctor had originally thought.

Since Gladys was thrilled to be graduating from hospice service her nurse, Tammy, thought that it would be nice to have a full-fledged graduation ceremony. The staff at the nursing home was excited to help out. One of the nursing home dining rooms was decorated in a graduation theme by her grand and great grandchildren. A special cake was baked by the hospice's staff and invitations made. For her Big Day, Gladys wore a cap and gown and was brought into the dining room while a recording of "Pomp and Circumstance" played. Nursing home staff, hospice staff and her family all cheered. Gladys was elated.

She received a Certificate of Graduation from the hospice's CEO, Denise Bauer RN, who said, "I wouldn't miss this event for the world. It's so wonderful to see such a large turnout of family and friends. And look at these great-grandchildren. This is what hospice is all about."

In a very unique way, another hospice patient was involved in, I guess you'd say, a "graduation situation" but with a pleasantly unexpected result. He was in his 70's. The social worker who was admitting him onto hospice asked, as our social workers ask every new admission, if he had any hopes, dreams, regrets, etc. Yes, in fact, he did have one regret. He said that during World War II, he dropped out of high school in his Senior Year so that he could join the military. He found out he wasn't medically qualified but he did go to work in one of the war factories.

After the War, he felt that he was too old to go back to high school. He eventually earned his GED (General Education Development) certificate. He got married and had a career. Now, all these years later, he was signing on to hospice and entering into what looked like his last stage of life. He regretted not receiving his high school diploma. So often the significance of an event is not known until it becomes a memory.

The regret that this man felt about not obtaining his high school diploma bothered the social worker. Soon she got the idea to write to the patient's old high school, which was in a major city several hundred miles away, to find out if they would consider awarding him a diploma, possibly an honorary one. After all, he dropped out of school for patriotic reasons and did complete his school work by earning his GED.

The high school thought that is was a great idea and agreed. Soon the patient had his diploma in hand. He was so proud. He showed his children and grandchildren. Everyone was happy for him including the hospice staff. And as they say in the TV infomercials, "But wait, there's more!"

Several weeks later he received a letter from his high school's alumni association. It was an invitation to his high school class reunion. He was included! Since he never graduated he was never registered as an alumnus and, therefore, had never received a class reunion invitation. He had long ago given up on the idea of attending his class reunion, even though he had been with the classmates through most of his school years. Besides, after several moves he lost track of everyone.

What a wonderful feeling it was for him to be included after all those years. That was the real reward. The simple gesture of being invited to the class reunion made the patient feel like he truly graduated with his classmates.

The hospice where I volunteer says that it celebrates life. It demonstrates that philosophy through efforts to help its patients celebrate the milestones of their life. We assist our patients in eliminating any regrets and helping them to enjoy the last stage of life.

Hospice knows that nothing is really over until you stop trying, and life is not over until a person gives up on living. My hospice encourages people on our service to appreciate and live life. Enjoy the little things because at some point you will look back and realize they were the big things.

~ I Love the Fair ~

I LOVE OUR county fair. One of the things that make it so important to me is that no matter what goes on in my life, the county fair will take place during the second week of October. That consistency, like the mail carrier stopping by every day, helps to keep my life in order.

The fair evolves, yet stays the same; young 4-h'ers grow up to be 4-H judges, cars that I remember as new are in the Demolition Derby, and the kids on the rides will someday bring their grandchildren to the fair. The ring toss where you win a cane will always be at the same location, the "Attention on the Midway!" announcements will never be replaced by email blasts, and harness racing will always be there. All of these things give me a secure feeling in a life of constant change and turmoil.

If you've lost someone close this past year, it's going to be a different fair this time. Noting will be the same, yet it will all be the same. If you're thinking about it, go to the fair. Consider going with someone who's also suffered a loss. Visit the places that bring back memories. Support each other as you share the good memories that a booth, a ride, or a certain building evokes. While there, it's okay to cry. It's good to cry and then laugh.

The county fair isn't just about fried food; it's also about emotional food. The county fair is about everything that is good in life. I love the fair.

~ Is it That Time Already? ~

THE HOLIDAY SEASON is the time of year when you hear a lot of good wishes, as well as a lot of complaining. You may also eat a lot of food and you may spend a lot of money. You may go to a lot of parties and go to church a lot (which is one of the best parts of the holiday season). There is definitely a lot going on during the holiday season.

If you have had someone close to you die this past year, you probably don't need a lot of anything except peace and quiet. It is a fact, though, that there is no way to get away from the "a lots." You will hear a lot about Thanksgiving and a lot about Christmas on TV, radio, and in most conversations. It seems like the retailers have been trying to stretch the holidays by starting with the relentless ads earlier and earlier. What can you do to get away from this over-activity?

If you have lost a loved one during this past year, the holidays will be different. Hospice understands the unique qualities of grief during the holidays and we are here to help. We know that there is no way to "get over it and be happy" during the holiday season if a loved one is no longer with you. I would like to offer some information that may be of help if you are dreading the holidays due to a loss.

When dealing with the holidays, there is what is known as the Five C's of Holiday Grief. If you have lost a loved one this past year, Thanksgiving, and Christmas, and maybe even New Year's Eve will be different. Even if you are having a hard time for any other reason during the holidays, the Five C's may offer a way to experience the holidays in a more tolerable manner.

The first "C" deals with **Communication.** Let people know what you need and what you can't handle. But also, be receptive to their concerns. If you don't want to go to a party because you may feel like a fifth wheel, then don't go. On the other hand, if you want to go to a party, try to drive yourself there. That way, if you feel overwhelmed you can excuse yourself and leave. If you have somebody drive you and you get tired early, ask if there is a room where you can be by yourself for a while. Tell the person who drove you that you are going to rest and will be back out soon.

Many grieving people will temporarily lose their tolerance for loud, busy family gatherings and can quickly be exhausted by the antics of small children. This is normal and will pass.

Also, as a way to make it through the holidays, the second "C" suggests that you **Cut back** on activities. Only do what you feel like doing. If putting up a lot of holiday decorations fills you with dread, pick and choose what is important for the holiday. Always ask yourself, "Would Christmas be the same without it?" If a big dinner seems overwhelming, have a potluck at someone else's house. You don't have to hang all the outside decorations this year or have a decoration in each room of the house, unless you want to. If this is your first year, it will be difficult. But each coming year will find you adding more of the things you liked about the holidays.

Change some of the things that you never liked about the holiday traditions. Did you always hate the inflated Santa that went in the front yard? Now you can change it. If there are parts of Christmas that were done because that's how they were always done, now you can change it. Some things that help are opening presents on a different night (Christmas night or day instead of Christmas Eve), going to church at a different time or going to a different church.

Celebrate! Yes, celebrate. It's important to remember why we celebrate Christmas. As your Christmas has been changed, this may be the time to redefine for yourself the meaning of Christmas. There will be tears and these are very normal. Now would be a great time to celebrate the life of your loved one with precious stories of previous holidays. Focusing on all the happy holidays that you had together may help you get through this one. This can be a wonderful time to share your memories and remembered stories, even if they bring tears.

And what would Thanksgiving or Christmas be without **Children**? The fifth "C" reminds you that children need stability and security all the time, but especially during the Thanksgiving and Christmas holidays. Ask children what they need to keep for Christmas traditions. What is important for them during the holidays? Ask them their opinion for changes that you'd like to make. Always remember that it takes many Christmases to be comfortable with new traditions and that many things change during the year. The first Christmas after the death will not be the way you will always do things for years to come.

I hope that, as you endure grieving through the holidays, you find the resolve to do what is best for you. I have found that the anticipation of a dreaded event is much worse than the actual event. Eventually your broken heart will begin to heal itself and your sadness will be interrupted by glimpses of joy and just maybe, a lot of joy.

During Thanksgiving and Christmas, I wish you peace and serenity. Everything is going to be okay.

~ ONE CARD TWICE ~

WHEN I BECAME a hospice volunteer, I never dreamed that there would be so many opportunities to serve. In one instance, I was asked by our chaplain if I would assist him as he facilitated a men's grief support group. He told me that all I needed to do was listen to the attendees. I figured that I could do that.

As it turned out, I'd known one of the attendees, "Kyle," on a casual basis for years. Our families went to the same church and his daughter was in my daughter's class. What brought Tom to the support group was that his wife, "Marilyn," died several years before. They were both in their mid-40's when she died. Kyle wasn't one for expressing himself too much and didn't speak very often during the group's discussions. One evening he came in to our group with a decidedly better outlook on life. He didn't want to say what caused the change for fear of people laughing at him. After a little coaxing, he proceeded to tell what happened that changed his outlook.

Kyle told me that it was important to know that since early childhood, Marilyn had saved every card that had been given to her. She had birthday cards, party invitations, Valentine's Day cards, Christmas cards, and cards for virtually any other occasion in her life. Marilyn continued this practice through her entire life, even saving the cards her children and husband received.

After almost 2 years following his wife's death, Kyle decided it was time to get rid of some of her belongings and move out of their big house. Tom felt he was doing okay, and besides, the kids had grown and were now on their own. While he was cleaning out a closet he came across four large, computer paper-type boxes full of all the cards his wife had saved. He called each of the children and asked if they wanted any of the cards that had originally been sent to them, but all declined. Since he didn't want any of them, he threw the boxes of cards away.

Getting rid of his wife's possessions had seemed like a good idea at the time but proved to be too much for him, so he decided to stay in the comfortable surroundings of their home. As the ensuing months dragged by, his grieving seemed to increase. He became very lonely and in his own words, "despondent." That's what brought him to our support group.

Several days before this particular support group, Tom got up and slowly prepared for the day ahead. Approaching the top of the steps to go down to the kitchen, as he had done every day for almost two years, he noticed something on the landing at the top of the steps. There, like a miniature pup tent, was a card.

He recognized it as the card that Marilyn had given to him years ago. There had been a rough spot in their marriage and they had separated. After they reconciled, she sent him a card in which she wrote that she realized they were soul mates. Marilyn promised that no matter how bad things got, she would always be there to comfort him. Tom told me at that moment he could feel a warmth come over him and his grief seemed to subside.

He had no explanation for the card at the top of the steps other than Marilyn gave him that one card twice…and this time he's keeping it. And, yes, he stopped coming to our men's grief support group.

~ One New Year's Resolution ~

FTER CHRISTMAS, MY thoughts are, "Okay, two holidays down and one to go." These three holidays are a sort of "Trifecta" of human concern. The focus of Thanksgiving is about thanking God for His many blessings of food, shelter, and family. The focus of Christmas is about celebrating His greatest gift to us, His only Son. Finally, the activities of New Year's focus on ourselves.

Many of us want to be entertained on New Year's Eve, but I also hear a lot of talk about New Year's Resolutions. The intent of a resolution is to improve ourselves in areas where we feel we are lacking. As a suggestion, before making any resolutions this year, say the long version of the Serenity Prayer.

"God, grant me the serenity to accept the things I cannot change, courage to change the things I can, and the wisdom to know the difference. Living one day at a time, enjoying one moment at a time, and accepting hardships as the pathway to peace. Taking, as Jesus did, this sinful world as it is, not as I would have it. Trusting that You will make all things right if I surrender to Your Will. So, I will be reasonably happy in this life and supremely happy with You forever in the next. Amen."

After saying that prayer, think about what is really important in your life. Write out your resolutions, then look them over. The first resolution must be to accept yourself as you are. Remember, God didn't make any mistakes. By accepting yourself as you are, you will gain serenity and then everything will work out just fine.

~ Oscar ~

I T'S IMPORTANT TO remember that in the last stage of a person's life everything in the household is in a stage of upheaval and everyone in the family is affected. This is especially true for pets. Sensing that something is wrong with their owner, coupled with the change in the old routine, can upset a pet.

My first experience with dogs grieving occurred with one of my earlier assignments. This story took place during the 1990's. A few things have changed since then, but during that time the hospice where I volunteer requested that the patient-contact volunteers assist in the bereavement follow up of their patient's family. In this instance, while I was visiting the widow three months after her husband died, I noticed that her dog, a dachshund named Oscar, was carrying a flannel shirt in his mouth when I entered the home.

The little guy had become a friend of mine during the months that I visited his owner, so we were glad to see each other. He put down the shirt and excitedly licked my face. The patient's wife told me that Oscar had been sleeping in his owner's chair since the day her husband died. She added that Oscar carries her husband's flannel shirt in his mouth wherever he goes.

Oscar seemed to exemplify what has been said about grief – that grief is love with nowhere to go. That seems especially true with dogs, the one who was always there for us. They can't express their grief to anyone. Where can he go for comfort? I don't know.

~ People Are the Important Part ~

WHEN I CONVERSE with patients and their families who are on hospice service during the Holidays there are many stories of Christmas past. In the over twenty years that I have been associated with hospice I don't remember any of those stories being about the fabulous Christmas gifts that someone bought for them. If there was any mention about gifts, the discussion was about gifts that were made for them by a friend or family member, not bought. That tells me that Christmas isn't about gifts. (OK, I guess a few mentioned the gorgeous diamond ring they received.)

For some, the next Christmas might not look like it's going to be a good one. Maybe there has been a loss of someone close, or maybe the loss of employment, or maybe it could be a case of the holiday blues. With the annual overdoing of Christmas movies and TV shows you will no doubt see a lot of sentimental hogwash, if I may be blunt. Although it's nice to fantasize that no one can live up to the perfect family celebrations that are portrayed.

Remember that the Christmas story, the original one, is about survival. The story unfolds when Joseph and his pregnant wife, Mary, had to make a difficult journey to their home town to register for the census. Because of the number of people arriving in their home town of Bethlehem there were no available rooms in which they could spend the night. As a result, they had to stay in a barn where the Baby Jesus was eventually born. Since they were in a barn the newborn Jesus was placed in the animals' food trough, a manger. Seemed like everything that could go wrong was going wrong.

I've learned never to ask, "What else could go wrong?" because something else always can. In the story of the birth of Jesus something else did go wrong. The ruler, King Herrod, heard of the "Newborn King" being born in his kingdom and was worried that he might lose his crown. So he ordered all infant males in his kingdom killed. Joseph, Mary, and the newborn Jesus had to escape to another country. Not an easy task for a newborn infant and his mother who was in no condition to travel.

But the story of Joseph and Mary and the birth of Jesus is also a story about peace, a peace that calms and comforts. And it's a story of love. We've all heard the carolers singing about peace on Earth and goodwill to men.

When I think of how the emphasis on buying Christmas gifts has caused society to drift from focusing on the true significance of the day, I am reminded of a story I read a long time ago. It was about a junior high school teacher whose class was getting fidgety in anticipation of their approaching Christmas break. The teacher knew he had to give the students a quick activity to try to get their minds off the approaching vacation. As a way to keep the students distracted, the teacher asked them to get out two sheets of paper. He then asked them to list the names of the other students in the room on those two sheets on the paper and to leave a space between each name.

He asked them to think of the nicest thing they could say about each of their classmates and write it down. As the teacher had hoped, it took the remainder of the class period for everyone to finish their assignment. As the students left the room, each one handed the papers in. Many were smiling, some weren't, but the main goal was reached; every one of them had calmed down.

Over the weekend the teacher wrote down the name of each student on a separate sheet of paper, and listed what everyone else had said about that individual. On Monday, he gave each student his or her list. Before long, the entire class was smiling, "Really?" was whispered. "I never knew that meant anything to anyone!" said another. "I didn't know others liked me so much."

The teacher felt good and was mildly surprised by everyone's happy reaction to reading what their classmates wrote about them. After that class, no one ever mentioned those papers again. The years went by and the students graduated. But that was not the end of it.

A few years after this particular class graduated, the parents of one of his students called the teacher. They said that their son, Ken, had been killed in Vietnam and that since the teacher had been his son's favorite teacher they asked him if he would attend the funeral. The teacher did attend. After the burial, there was a fellowship lunch at the home of Ken's parents and most of his former classmates attended.

After lunch Ken's mother and father approached the teacher and said they had something the teacher might be interested in. Ken's father took a wallet out of his pocket and told the teacher that they had found it on Ken when he was killed. "We thought that you might recognize it."

Opening the wallet, Ken's dad carefully removed two worn pieces of notebook paper that had obviously been taped, folded, and refolded many times. The teacher knew instantly that the papers were the ones on which he had listed all the good things each of Ken's classmates had said about him. Ken's mom thanked the teacher for doing that. She knew that her son had treasured it.

Ken's classmates started to gather around them. One of the students smiled rather sheepishly and said, "I still have my list. It's in the top drawer of my desk at home."

"I put mine in my wedding album," said another classmate.

Yet another said, "I have mine too. It's in my diary."

One of the classmates reached into her pocketbook, took out her wallet and showed her worn and frazzled list to the group. Still another classmate said that she keeps her list with her at all times. It sounded like the whole class had saved their list. A simple act had such an unexpectedly profound effect on all those students. To me, that's what the Christmas story is about; a simple, profound act of love.

This Christmas you may want to try to avoid over-doing it. As hospice patients and families have told me, people are the important part of Christmas, not the gifts.

~ People Know We Care ~

THERE IS A truism in life that says, "People don't care how much you know until they know how much you care." What reminded me of that quote was that I recently read a short article about Jim Towey. A high-level lawyer, Mr. Towey served as one of President George Bush's Senior Advisers. He was also a friend of Mother Teresa and volunteered as her legal counselor. In order to learn more about Mother Teresa's work, Jim Towey visited her Home for the Dying in Calcutta, India during the 1980's.

Through this association with her and by actually seeing firsthand the work that she did he was struck that, in that haven in the Third World, "...the dying people's hands were held, their pain was managed, and they weren't alone." In contrast, he said that "...in the First World, (i.e.; the so called advanced countries) you see a lot of medical technology, but people die in pain, and alone."

The medical staff of a hospice has a lot of medical knowledge and they are technologically savvy, but that doesn't seem to impress a terminally ill person's family. At the hospice where I volunteer, the many thank you cards we receive never say how glad they were that some of our staff graduated at the top of their class. None of the cards mentioned how many letters some of our staff have behind their name. They will, however, mention that one of our home health aides sat in the living room to talk to a patient's spouse for a half hour, or that one of our doctors stopped by their house to see how their Dad was feeling.

What is important is that those who have experienced hospice know we care.

~ She Left as She Came ~

WE ENTER THIS world with no earthly concerns or earthly possessions. And I've heard many times that one of the pathways to peace and serenity is let go of earthly concerns and earthly possessions. Not long ago, the hospice where I volunteer signed a pragmatic woman onto our service who very poignantly confirmed those two statements. Her illness was incurable and instead of fighting it to the bitter end (and have people proud of her for doing so), she decided to sign on to hospice service and enjoy, as much as possible, her last stage of life.

Once settled into her new routine of living and not going anywhere for another treatment, she decided to give her valuables to her children, allowing her to see their reaction rather than leaving the items in her will to be divvied up later. After she gave away those items, she arranged for an auction company to sell her remaining items, sold her house, and moved in with one of her children. She was now free of any earthly possessions and ready to meet her Creator.

The only problem was that her Creator was not ready to meet her. As often happens when someone signs on to hospice service soon enough after the six-month prognosis, her health improved. No longer appropriate for hospice, she signed off of service. She moved in with her son and, as I heard later, lived a very happy, carefree life with no earthly concerns or earthly possessions.

Time passed and she eventually signed back on to hospice, dying in her sleep the next day. This woman truly left this life the same way that she entered – with nothing and not a care in the world.

~ SINGLE BELLS ~

A FEW YEARS ago, I had a hard time coming up with a "true meaning of Christmas" column. I confided this to my writing mentor who suggested that maybe someone needed to watch "A Charlie Brown Christmas" one more time. I did and she was right.

In that classic, Charlie Brown tells Linus that even with all the festivities of the season, he still feels depressed. Many of us feel that way. This is the season when we think that we have to be happy. But if you've lost someone, don't you dread this time of year? You know everyone expects you to put on your happy face. The trouble is, it's not just a single holiday. We've just finished one tradition-filled holiday and here comes another one. It can be too much. Understand that you are not only grieving your loved one, but also grieving the old holidays that are now changed forever. Your family portrait has been permanently changed and so have the holidays.

Remember when the Peanuts gang gathered for play practice and looked at Charlie Brown's pathetic little tree? They all laughed except Linus. He had had enough. He went on stage and recited the Christmas story from Luke 2:8-14. After listening to Linus, Charlie Brown realized that he didn't have to let the commercialism, the parties, or the expectations of others ruin his Christmas. You don't either.

Hold on to the happy memories of Christmas Past. Keep Christmas Present simple and serene. Know that Christmas Future will be new and wonderful. Everything's going to be okay.

~ Support Afterwards ~

EACH HOSPICE IS unique. What makes hospice in general somewhat uniform is that all hospices must adhere to Medicare guidelines in order to receive reimbursement. The hospice where I volunteer takes the initiative to be available to the entire community, and in more ways than just comforting the terminally ill and their family. My hospice is available to anyone who is grieving a loss. And by "anyone," I'm including both adults and children.

Among the many avenues of grief support that the hospice where I volunteer offers for adults are two types of support groups; a structured six-week support group and a weekly group. The six-week group is somewhat structured and each week deals with a different subject, such as anger, or depression. We ask that those wanting to attend this group register for it. There is no charge to attend, but we need to know how many to expect so that we have enough booklets and supplies. The weekly group is a walk-in type open discussion support group. Again, there is no charge for these groups.

Grief can isolate a person. Being alone may just seem easier. To offer a way out of isolation for those making the journey through grief, we offer our monthly social group. This is a somewhat loose-knit group who are progressing through the grief journey and desire to get out in public more. They meet for lunch at an area restaurant once a month. Just to make life interesting, the location for each meeting varies month to month.

As stated before, all the grief activities my hospice offers are open to anyone, of any age, and at no charge. There are myriad reasons for someone to be in the throes of grief. We know that some people prefer to fight an illness to the bitter end. Fighting a serious illness is a very personal matter and it's their choice. Then comes the grief. And should someone be thrust into grief as the result of a sudden death, grieving can be especially difficult. The sudden death may be due to an accident, an overdose, a suicide, an illness, or a host of other reasons. We offer our support to everyone.

Support groups may be appropriate when you are grieving, but suppose friends and family don't see a need for you to grieve? Maybe there is more to the story and they just don't understand. An example of such a situation may be the death of an ex-spouse. Friends and family might assume that you are relieved that the ex-spouse is gone. In one of the support groups a woman was talking about why she was attending the support group. She said her friends told her that technically she shouldn't be grieving the death of her ex-husband. After all, she initiated the divorce. One of the others in the group quickly asked, "Since when is grief controlled by a technicality?" I couldn't have answered it better.

The value of a support group allows people to know that they are not alone. It's the one place to be understood and find hope after a devastating loss. And hope is tremendous progress for someone who once felt hopeless. Support groups help you to understand that what you are experiencing is normal.

In another situation, a man was in a support group because his cat died. On the surface that didn't seem like a reason to grieve. He said that he was too embarrassed to tell his family about his feelings. But as he continued, he told how he brought the cat home from a shelter when his wife was very sick. The cat was such a comfort to her, plus knowing that the cat was a "rescue" made his wife feel good inside.

Naturally, when his wife eventually passed the man grieved, but not to the extent that his family anticipated. Evidently, the cat became a physical part of his wife's memory in which he found comfort and something he could literally hold on to. But years later when the cat died, he truly began to grieve for his wife. It looked to his family as if he was grieving more for the cat than he did for his wife. The animal's end was the beginning of his real grief for his wife. He felt the need to come to the support group. As it turned out, another attendee in the group had a very similar experience.

After attending a grief support group for a period of time, people have told me that they began to notice the similarities in others in the group and not the differences. Although each person's grief response is unique, there are the three "N's" of grief that everyone will at some point go through and understand: Grief is Normal, Natural and Necessary.

The hospice where I volunteer has a grief center with meeting rooms of various sizes for individual or family counseling, for counselling children, and there is a very large room for meetings, celebrations, and children's grief camp activities.

You'll notice that I've mentioned children's grief and counselling grieving children. As children change from early childhood on through the teenage years, they continue to change physically and emotionally and, consequently, need special grief support. Our children's grief program, PALS (Peace, Acceptance, Love, Support) is a highly-acclaimed children's grief program. Our grief center is the perfect location for our PALS program with plenty of room to allow the children to actively work through their grief.

No one understands the depth of your grief but you. Someone in a support group once said to me that he wished Heaven had visiting hours. Sadly, it doesn't but hospice is always available to listen. Everything is going to be okay.

~ Survivors of a Suicide Death ~

T HE HOSPICE WHERE I volunteer offers grief support for anyone affected by a death. These deaths can be from an accident, heart attack, stroke, drug overdose, and the one no one really ever talks about, suicide. The difference with these deaths as opposed to a "normal" death is the trauma the family and friends suffer afterwards. The "why's" and "I-should-have's" can be overwhelming.

Survivors of a suicide death are the most overlooked grievers. The stigma and taboo that go along with suicide seemingly don't give them the right to grieve, so they often hold their feelings inside. In reality, suicide is just another word for death.

After any death, there are five domains of grief-related stress. These five domains are:

- The physical domain which includes exhaustion, headaches, and stomach aches.
- The emotional domain, which may include overwhelming and uncontrollable tears, as well as intense reactions.
- The cognitive domain in which the griever is unable to concentrate or stay focused.
- The social domain manifests when remaining relationships just require energy that the griever doesn't have.
- And the spiritual domain in which the griever is questioning the meaning and purpose of life.

These five domains are primary in all grieving processes, whether the death was due to trauma or was a "normal" death.

The hospice where I volunteer and most, if not all other hospices, offer support and comfort to anyone seeking it. Hope is found here.

~ WHAT ABOUT THE YOUNG PEOPLE? ~

MY EXPERIENCE HAS been that when someone thinks of hospice, they associate us with older people dying. The truth is that hospice cares for anyone who is dying, regardless of their age. And what you also may not know is that we comfort anyone who has experienced a loss, regardless of their age. The hospice where I volunteer offers grief support through our weekly grief support groups, and through our structured six-week program. But don't think that grief support is only for "older" people.

Many hospices, including the one where I volunteer, offer free grief support services for the young people, the children. Children are constantly developing, and the loss of a special person may deeply influence a child's development. Many hospices, including mine, offer a feature that often helps young people deal with an approaching loss, i.e., anticipatory grief. These kids may range in age from as young as four years old through the teenage years.

Why something special for children, especially those as young as four or five years old? They are not old enough to realize what is going on, are they? Yes, they are. Children do not grieve the same way that adults do and it may not be easily recognizable. Sometimes what looks like play may be the way the child is processing their grief.

If you have experienced a loss of any sort in your family, think of hospice. Your heart aches for the adults, but what about the young people?

~ ATTENTION AND RESPECT ~

THERE IS A saying in the funeral industry that a good funeral gets the dead where they need to go and the living where they need to be. Part of what hospice can do is to get the living where they need to be, from an emotional point of view. We accomplish this by taking the time to learn what the person on service and their family really cares about.

While at a memorial service, a woman told me that her mother, who had been on our service, wanted to be cremated so no traditional funeral arrangements had been made. One of the benefits of Calling Hours at a funeral is that the family and friends get to see the deceased one last time. And if I can be gentle about it, the deceased look more presentable at a funeral home then they did immediately after they died.

The hospice nurse and the family were there when the woman on service died. Knowing this would be the last time that the grown daughter would get to see her mom, Heidi, the hospice nurse, quickly got to work. Heidi asked several aides to help her bathe and dress the mom's body in nice clothes. They put clean linens on the bed, combed the woman's hair and put make-up on her. It meant so much to the daughter to see the attention and respect given to her mom and (indirectly) to the family, even after the woman had died.

In doing so, Heidi helped the daughter to emotionally arrive at exactly where she needed to be.

~ AVOID CLICHÉS LIKE THE PLAGUE ~

EVERY ONCE IN a while, I like to put a little levity into what I write. So, for this short piece, I thought that I might go out on a limb and lighten things up a bit. As a rule of thumb, I keep things plain and simple but I thought maybe I could use a few clichés to make this sound like an April Fools' essay – not the same old song and dance.

Variety is the spice of life. Who knows, maybe a little change will do me good. I'll try to keep it short and sweet, although that might be easier said than done. Being under the gun I worked like a dog on this book, with their subjects being all over the map.

Even after all this time, I think I'm still at the tip of the iceberg writing about the goodness of hospice. This isn't rocket science, but I do try to think outside the box, leaving no stone unturned. I often use patient-related experiences such as the conversation of the doctor telling his patient, "You have one foot in the grave. Further tests will determine if it's the right or left."

If in a crisis, you may have the feeling of being at the end of your rope. But when choosing hospice, the ball is in your court. Not to gloss it over, just know that when push comes to shove, there's always a glimmer of hope and hope springs eternal.

Last but not least, this tongue-in-cheek essay was barely completed in the nick of time, so I hope it looks good on paper. And I always proofread to make sure I don't _____ any words out.

~ Cab Ride to Hospice ~

IN AN EFFORT to pay my way through college, I drove a Yellow Cab in Dayton, Ohio during part of 1972. Taxi cabs were still an important part of the cityscape in that year. My cab was #30 and that has been my lucky number ever since. Those seven months behind the wheel of a taxi exposed me to every facet of life. And as I look back on my life, one fare that took 20 minutes from start to finish, eventually brought me to my last career position – volunteering and working for a local hospice.

On a very drizzly, dismal, dark evening in late February, I was dispatched to the Emergency Room of Miami Valley Hospital to pick up a fare. Since the location of a hospital's Emergency Room is familiar to everyone, that was where most taxi related hospital pick-ups were. Emergency Room fares were always interesting because I never knew if the fare would be a banged-up Emergency Room patient being released, a staff member needing a ride home, or any of a myriad of reasons someone needed a ride.

As I pulled up, a small, frail woman probably in her 80's approached my cab. I got out and assisted her into the back seat. Her address was on Xenia Avenue, just east of downtown. Since we were heading to an older part of the city I asked her about the neighborhood, how long she had lived there, etc. I always enjoy hearing about the "good 'ol days." She talked for a bit about the neighborhood, then gently turned the conversation towards me. I told her that I was recently married and that my wife had been a nurse for about a year.

"Oh, you two have your whole life in front of you." She sounded so happy and excited.

Then, as she gazed out the side window of the cab, she said that she had been at the hospital visiting her husband of 63 years and that he was very sick. I wasn't sure how to respond. But after a few seconds of quiet, she continued talking, almost wistfully, about her husband and their life together. Being newly married, I found it fascinating.

"His nurse said that he wasn't doing very well and that he needed his rest. Someone came in and said that visiting hours are over and that maybe I should go home and get some rest, too." Talking softly, as if to herself, she said, "He's going to die tonight, I know it. They wouldn't let me stay." I thought to myself, "After an entire life together, on a day that was just as important as their wedding day, why did the hospital staff send her home? Why separate them when their need for each other is so intense?"

I pulled up to their house, the house they moved into as young-marrieds so many years before. Low clouds and drizzle muffled the sounds of the city and dimly reflected the lights of downtown onto the small front yard. Hurrying around the cab, I opened the taxi's rear door for her and she slowly got out. I instinctively put my arm around her and walked her up to the front porch.

She gave me the house key and I let her in. She wished me and my wife a happy life together and as I turned to leave she embraced me, pressed her head in my shoulder and started to sob. "He was such a good man. I'm going to miss him…I'm so scared." Caught off guard, I held her for a bit. I did not want to leave her.

Again she said, "He's going to die tonight. I know it. Why wouldn't they let me stay?" Again, I had no reply. She turned, went in, and I stood there as the door closed. After a moment, I turned and took a few steps toward my cab. I stopped. My bottom lip started to quiver and my eyes moistened. Gazing back at the dark silhouette of her house I realized her life was ending, mine was beginning. It was as if she had passed the baton of life to me.

A lot has changed in the medical field since 1972, but the change hasn't just been in technology or pharmaceuticals. There has also been a change, albeit a small one, in the thinking on the part that the family plays when dealing with a serious illness. Through the hospice philosophy, we are turning back from medical invincibility to reality.

When I think of that woman I picked up from Miami Valley Hospital, I think how different it would have been had hospice come to America by that time. Hospice care has brought some common sense into what modern thinking had turned into a clinical event – the end of life. Common sense, or maybe I should say "hospice sense," tells me that the woman's husband did not need rest. Rest for what? He needed his wife and she needed him. She needed to be with him and to comfort him. Couldn't the hospital staff have bent the rules just a little for her? All these years later, I still think of her. Little did I know that that short fare would eventually bring me to hospice.

Twenty-five years later, in January of 1997, I saw an ad in the paper about hospice seeking volunteers and instinctively knew that I had to do it. I didn't know much about hospice then but I did know that hospice care focused on people. That it encouraged family and friends to gather when someone was approaching the end of their life, and didn't send family home to "get some rest." In fact, many times at the hospice where I now volunteer, our staff has helped a spouse get in bed with their dying partner so that the one could comfort the other.

When I got back in my taxi that night, the dispatcher was calling my number. He had a pick up for me at the Galaxy Club on Linden Avenue…. It was a "go-go joint".… And life went on.

~ CHESTER CONSOLING ~

MANY VISITORS DON'T know that we have a resident cat, Chester, at the hospice house where I volunteer. And that is just fine with him. He arrived on his own one summer and has, at his discretion, been a part of the staff ever since.

When Chester was still "new in these parts," a woman was admitted to our facility for end-of-life care. As the woman was being brought in, her daughter followed as the nurse and aide accompanied the patient into her room. Chester quietly followed the entourage into the room and lay down at the daughter's feet. A fast friendship developed.

During this stage of life, the illness may not be the problem. The problem may be relationships, whether with family or with God. In this case, the mother and daughter had a few issues to work out and lengthy discussions took place in the room. Chester was always at the daughter's feet.

Several days after her arrival, the mother died. The daughter, of course, was upset and went to the Sun Room to be alone and cry. As she slumped into a chair to cry, Chester, who had followed her to the room, jumped onto her lap and began to meow softly. For almost an hour as the emotion ran its course, Chester held on, resting his head on her stomach and softly meowing.

That was the first time any of our staff saw Chester console anyone, but it's a scenario that is now seen more frequently. Everyone in my hospice is dedicated to comforting, even our cat.

~ Everyday War Stories ~

MY EXPERIENCE AS a hospice patient care volunteer has afforded me the privilege of getting to know veterans and to hear their war stories. Sometimes it was the first time they spoke of them and sometimes the family was tired of hearing them. Didn't matter, I'd listen. One patient who comes to mind had been a tail gunner on a B-17 in the European Theater during WWII. He said that it was fun until his third mission when a German fighter shot off part of his plane's tail, about a foot over his head. He told me that event brought up an interesting point – in a plane you fight until you or your enemy is killed. There is no place to hide.

A couple of my patients were veterans of Iwo Jima. Both patients were sullen and withdrawn. The only thing one patient would say about it was, "A bad place." At the other's funeral, only his wife, one child and I attended. Evidently, throughout his life he just couldn't leave Iwo behind.

A Navy veteran told me that his destroyer and a second one were assigned to zig-zag over the entire surface of Tokyo Bay just after Japan's surrender. Even though minesweepers had done their job, his ship's mission was to bump into any undetected, usually wooden, mines in the water, thus making the harbor safe for the "big wigs." The Navy wanted to make sure that the minesweepers didn't miss anything before the USS Missouri entered to accept the surrender of the Japanese. "That ought to make you feel important," my patient said with a wry smile.

Another patient showed me a stack of photos of a concentration camp that his company had liberated. Most disturbing were the photos of the piles of infant blankets, clothing and booties sorted by type of material.

For some, serving in the military has been a lifelong experience. Thank you, veterans.

~ We Don't Know Them All ~

I GRADUATED FROM SCHOOL in 1967. After graduation, some of us stayed close to the area but many went off to college or into the military. In early May of 1968, I received a phone call from a former classmate, "Did you hear about Dale?" Dale Hess was one of our high school classmates and was so well known that he became one of those one-name people such as "Michael" or "Cher." He had been class president, served on the student council, and seemed to excel in everything he did.

"Hear about Dale?" I replied.

All I knew was that he had enlisted in the Marines after high school. The caller told me that Dale had been killed in Vietnam and that his funeral would be in a few days. I was stunned. It may sound silly, but he was the first person I ever knew who got killed in a war. All I could think of was, of all people, why Dale? Not that anyone is better or worse than anyone else, but still, why Dale?!

In a class of about 210 students, everybody knew Dale Hess and everybody liked him. What impressed me in particular was that he was approachable and talked to everyone. He was almost a year older than I was, even though we were in the same grade. He was born in November while I was born the end of the following October. For a teenager, a year's difference in age can be huge. I remember having several long conversations with him in school. Those conversations have been part of the few fond memories I have of high school.

Several years ago, I visited the Vietnam Traveling Memorial Wall when it came to the Fairfield County Fairgrounds. I wanted to see Dale's name. There were some brochures at the display that explained The Wall. Yes, it's more than names on a wall. I learned that the names on "The Wall," as it has come to be known, are placed in the approximate order of death, beginning in the center, and continuing to the right point (as you look at it) of the Wall. The first person listed as killed in Vietnam is on the top left corner of panel 1E on the right of the center seam.

Then the names continue in their chronological sequence to the right point. On the far left point, all the way over to the opposite end of The Wall, the names continue in their chronological sequence. The names continue to the right, ending with the last person killed in the Vietnam War on the bottom of the panel left of the center seam. Therefore, at the center seam of The Wall names of the first killed are next to the names of the last killed. It is a symbolic closing of the wound the Vietnam War opened in our country.

While I was at the Vietnam Traveling Memorial Wall display, I decided to look up the name of another classmate whom I heard might have been killed in Vietnam. He'd left school after about 2 years and I lost track of him. His name was Mike. He always seemed nervous and got into trouble a few times at school. From what I remember, Mike also had problems at home. We didn't have all the student services and counsellors during that era so if a student had problems, they had to tough it out if they could. At some point, he transferred to another high school. I heard that Mike joined the Army during the winter of my senior year.

Sadly, I did find Mike's name in the listing of names on the Vietnam Traveling Memorial Wall. After I got home I looked up information about Dale and Mike on a website that gives brief information about how each person earned a place on The Wall. I found out that Mike's tour in Vietnam began on June 13, 1967 and he became a casualty less than two weeks later on June 26 in Quang Ngai Province. Dale's name was located several panels further to the right because he was killed about 10 months after Mike. Through the website, I found that Dale began his tour on November 28, 1967 and his casualty date was April 30, 1968. He was killed in Quang Tri Province. Two completely different men met the same fate.

Researching the Vietnam Memorial in Washington D.C., I learned that there is a memorial in the Vietnam Memorial Park in Washington D.C. for those who weren't killed in combat but died later, as a direct result of the Vietnam War. It's the "In Memory" plaque. The In Memory Plaque Memorial was dedicated on

November 10, 2004 to honor those who died prematurely because of war related illness. Among the eligible diagnoses were Agent Orange poisoning and Post Traumatic Stress Disorder (PTSD).

In the 1970's one of my coworkers, John, had a good, secure job in the growing company that employed us. He was married with several children, volunteered in the community, etc. One day after work, we were sitting in the break room discussing the day over a cup of coffee. Both of us loved it there and on many late afternoons we would sit and talk about the day.

This time he told me in a matter-of-fact tone of voice that he had just turned in his resignation. John also said he had filed for divorce and was planning to leave the area, the area where he was born and raised. I thought he was kidding. He then got up, we shook hands and he left. I honestly did not believe that he was serious. Next morning the Personnel Manager told me John was using his sick-days allotment for his last two weeks. He literally got up and left the life he was living. It was as if he had died emotionally. I later learned that what he did was somewhat common for those with PTSD.

Hospice empathizes with veterans because we employ quite a few. For veterans on our service, we provide a pinning ceremony and other forms of recognition. In particular, the hospice where I volunteer offers grief support to anyone suffering from a loss, even if their loved one was a combat casualty. We know that families of combatants pay such a high price.

Memorial Day is a time to reflect on the sacrifices made by regular people like Dale, Mike, and John. Stories similar to theirs can be told relative to any war. If you can spare a few minutes, stop by any cemetery and, if nothing else, trim the grass from around the base of a veteran's gravestone. I read somewhere that we don't know them all but we owe them all.

~ Veteran's Day ~

NOVEMBER 11 IS Veteran's Day. Most of the media attention given to Veteran's Day seems to deal with war. However, the majority of veterans have not been in combat. My uncle, for example, spent World War II in Ft. Thomas, Kentucky. It was about 5 miles from his home.

When enlisting, no one knows where they will end up. The Recruiter may promise the prospective candidate a certain job classification and a certain area of the country, but once in, there is no guarantee, and no apologies from anyone. While serving under Patton, my Dad said he heard the sentence, "You're in the Army now," many times when duties or plans were abruptly changed.

I heard it explained once that life is like a train. People who sign up for military service are taken off the train and stay at the station while the train of life continues. When veterans are discharged from the service, they get back on the train but everyone in their life is way ahead of them, their lives have continued on uninterrupted. New relationships may have been formed, and old friends may have changed. The veterans were taken out of circulation and now must start where they left off. That is a tremendous sacrifice no matter what they did in the service or where they served.

Whether serving in combat or serving in Ft. Thomas, Ky., anyone who has served in the military deserves our respect for the sacrifice that they made. Thank you, veterans.

~Even a Little Fawn ~

THE WOMAN HAD been non-communicative and sleeping long hours for several days when one of my hospice's volunteers, Janet, came to visit her at the hospice house. The weather was perfect, so Janet helped the hospice house aide bring her out to the back patio, in her hospital bed, to enjoy the weather.

As Janet closed the hospice facility's patio door, she noticed a deer and her fawn observing everything from the edge of the woods fifty feet away. Janet softly told the woman that a mother deer and her fawn wanted to visit. The woman very slowly moved her hand through the bedrail. Janet thought that she did this possibly to let her arm dangle in order to better feel the gentle breeze.

Janet noticed that the mother and fawn were slowly approaching. The little one continued onto the patio while the mother stayed back. The fawn, leaning against the bedrail, walked the length of the woman's bed gently letting the woman's hand glide along its head. Janet noticed the sleeping woman faintly smile. The fawn then scampered back to its mother. Janet stood transfixed. A moment later the woman took a deep breath, as if giving a sigh of relief, then died.

My hospice's facility is not on a busy street. In my heart, I believe that the location was Divine Intervention so that all His creation, even a little fawn, could help comfort not only those on our hospice service, but also their families, our staff, and volunteers.

~ COMPASSIONATE, CREATIVE PEOPLE ~

ONE THING ABOUT working at my hospice is that I'm not just another pretty face around here. Hospice is well known for its compassionate care of the ill person and their family because of the quality of people we hire. When a person becomes a part of the hospice staff, either as a paid staff member or a volunteer, they are given a degree of free space to use their creativity to help our patients.

Sometimes this creativity results in a new therapy for our hospice to offer to its patients. Our Touch Therapy, Pet Therapy, Music Therapy, and Massage Therapy were a direct result of our volunteers wanting to use their skills to help our patients. Our P.A.L.S. program for grieving children and our company-sponsored fundraisers are also the result of volunteer and staff creativity.

Our United Way Campaign, that assists with bereavement activities, is successful because of the creativity of a committee of staff members who run the campaign. Hospice receives many compliments regarding the amazing care that is provided to the people on our service, and their families. They are complemented for the willingness of all our staff, paid and volunteer, to do what needs doing when it needs to be done.

In fact, my hospice's office staff has many members who began their career with us as volunteers. They felt so strong about being associated with hospice that they were willing to first give of themselves in one of the various volunteer avenues. As we grew, some joined us as paid staff.

I think that hospice is always looking for people with a compassionate heart. We don't need just a pretty face.

~ OH, I DON'T WANT TO HEAR ABOUT THAT ~

I WAS IN the dining room of a senior citizen apartment building preparing to speak to a group of residents when a wheelchair-bound woman rolled in. She asked what I was doing and I told her that I was preparing to speak to the residents about hospice.

"Oh, I don't want to hear about that crap!" she said and turned her wheelchair to leave. I showed her that I had brought homemade cookies and lemonade from our hospice facility so she decided to stay. I might point out that she stayed afterward to further discuss what we do at hospice. That always happens.

Should you want to learn about hospice care, most hospices offer speakers to make presentations. Personally, I have spoken to a wide variety of groups from a few people in a card club to over 500 employees at a distribution center. Topics may range from general hospice information to presentations on paperwork at the end of life. Your group might be interested in having a hospice chaplain present on end-of-life spiritual issues. Often, one of the hospice's medical staff will present to the medical community.

Neither my hospice nor most other hospices charge for this service. If you, your group, or organization would like a speaker for a club meeting or any type of gathering, please call your area hospice. You may be like the woman in the wheelchair and stay late to learn more.

~ Normal, Everyday People ~

HOSPICE IS KNOWN for giving extraordinary care. We accomplish this extraordinary level of care through a team approach in caring for the person on service. I'm not kidding when I say we use the team approach, because each patient will have a doctor, nurse, social worker, aide, chaplain, and the option of a volunteer on their care team.

A volunteer is a part of the team?! Yes, the normal, everyday people who volunteer are an integral part of the care team. In fact, Medicare requires that volunteers must provide day-to-day administrative and/or direct patient care in an amount that, at a minimum, equals 5% of the total patient care hours of all paid hospice employees and contract staff. Medicare also requires that hospice volunteers be used in defined roles and under the supervision of a hospice employee. Regarding the hospice where I volunteer, that employee is the Director of Volunteers. It's a little-known fact that the hospice movement in the United States was started by volunteer doctors, nurses, and various other medical and nonmedical people.

Volunteers by their nature are deeply involved because they want to be involved. They are from the general population and are not on the care team for any purpose other than to help where needed. They bring a calmness and normalcy to hospice and especially the people on hospice service.

The training to become a volunteer is not stressful. Surprisingly, much of the training is actually enjoyable. My hospice has always been a relaxed, family-focused organization and our volunteer training program reflects that. The volunteer training classes generally last for about three hours per session and, as a rule, are held one session per week for six weeks. The size of the training class may range anywhere from five people to around twenty. The training classes expose the new volunteers to many areas of hospice volunteering that they may not have known about, including: patient care, fundraising, office work, or public outreach. The new volunteers are encouraged to volunteer in an area that interests them.

Not only do we teach them about being a volunteer, but they have also taught us a thing or two. As the volunteer gains experience in our organization, they realize that they may be able to help us in new ways. In fact, several of our therapies are the result of a volunteer seeing a need and using their knowledge and talent to develop a new therapy for the benefit of the people under our care.

An example of something initiated by one of our volunteers is the children's grief program, PALS (Peace, Acceptance, Love, Support). It was developed by a volunteer who had extensive experience in the public-school system. She realized that some of the children who were having problems in school were actually grieving the loss of someone. Her experience as an educator helped her develop the children's grief program that is now available throughout our three-county service area. It's amazing what one volunteer can do.

There are many areas of hospice in which to volunteer but the area that seems to generate the most apprehension, or fear, to someone considering being a volunteer at a hospice is that of patient-contact volunteer. Don't worry, no volunteer is asked to do anything that they do not want to do. Personally, I felt called to be a patient-contact volunteer but all volunteers have the option to decline that area of volunteering.

The primary purpose of the hospice patient-contact volunteer is to offer respite, or a rest, to the caregiver. Generally, the volunteer will stay with the patient while the caregiver runs errands, attends functions, or just takes a nap. My hospice puts a limit of 4 hours per volunteer visit. If more time is needed, a second volunteer comes in after 4 hours to relieve the first volunteer.

In one instance, we had a very young person on service staying for a few days at our hospice house. What led to the child's stay was that her mother was only taking short naps for fear of not being awake if her child needed her. The hospice Director of Volunteers put out a call for volunteers to sit at the child's bedside while the mother got some sleep. Pairs of volunteers, many of them husband and wife teams, maintained a steady through-the-night vigil at the little one's bedside so the mother could rest. Every two hours, new volunteers came in to relieve the other volunteers.

By the time a family signs a loved one onto a hospice's service, they are at their wits' end. The importance of a volunteer is that he/she may be the only person on the hospice team who doesn't have an agenda or a specific purpose. Therefore, the volunteer is non-threatening and able to help the family in whatever capacity they request. The volunteer's scheduled visits usually continue for as long as the patient is on service.

Something that technology can't change is that life begins with family and ends with family. Through compassionate care provided by hospice staff, and its volunteers, the end of life can be a return to personal family time, a time before the modern age turned dying into a medical event. I hope that I have helped to remove some of the mystery behind what hospice's volunteers do. Through ordinary people, hospice gives extraordinary care.

~ Pet Therapy ~

EVEN THE LOWLY goldfish won at the county fair that is here today and gone tomorrow has a positive effect on the owner. For most of us pets are, or were, a part of the family. Many studies have shown that animals, especially family pets, are a source of comfort in a crisis. Hospice understands the importance of pets to humans.

One of the many comfort therapies that is offered by the hospice where I volunteer is given by, shall I say, our two "four legged therapists." That therapy is Pet Therapy and it truly works wonders. Our therapy dogs are currently Brinkli and Oscar. They have helped our families find serenity and comfort when their world is coming apart. The dogs provide an emotional outlet that does not require thought, concentration, or talking. They have no fear of rejection, they don't care how the patient looks, nor do they have any preconceived notion about social status. The therapy dogs are just glad to visit. They softly convey the message, "I understand."

After experiencing a visit by either Oscar or Brinkli, people have said that they were just visited by angels in a dog's body. Everyone who has been visited by these "furry angels" feels calmed and reassured. And it's not just dogs that have such a good effect on people. Any pet whether a bird, cat, or fish offers stress relief. Simply watching fish in an aquarium has a soothing affect…. but so far, we haven't found anyone willing to lug an aquarium around to anyone on our service .

~ Dogs Feel it Too ~

A T THE HOSPICE where I volunteer, a patient had a friendly, outgoing dog. This furry family member welcomed each hospice staff member at the front door when they visited the patient's home. Through all the visits by the hospice staff, this canine member of the family remained friendly, almost happy. It was almost like she was saying, "You are here to help, aren't you?" Each wag of her tail was a "Thank you!"

One evening the hospice nurse was called to the home because the patient's Hour had come. As the nurse entered the home, she noticed that she was not greeted by the dog. Instinctively, the nurse knew something had happened. Sure enough, the patient had passed a little while earlier. As the nurse was consoling the spouse, she heard a high-pitched whimper and noticed that the dog was curled up behind her owner's favorite recliner. If dogs cry, she was crying.

This incident reminded me of how the caring hospice personnel are concerned with all who are affected by the illness and the passing, even pets. The fact that the nurse mentioned the dog's reaction to the death in her report emphasized her concern.

For me, this was one of many episodes of dogs feeling the pangs of loss while I've been involved with hospice. Although I haven't read any studies on the subject, I've witnessed and was made aware of too many stories about dogs grieving to doubt that, yes, dogs feel it too.

~ Thanks, Dad ~

I REMEMBER SEEING a particular "For Better or For Worse" cartoon in the Comics Section of the paper. It was a five-box comic that featured an older man and his grown son leaning on the porch railing, gazing into the night sky. The first two boxes simply show the two men silently gazing. In the third box, the dad says, "I'm proud of you, son. You're doing a good Job" In the fourth box, the dad has his hand on his son's shoulder and the son replies, "Thanks, Dad." In the fifth box, there is a thought bubble over their heads with both thinking the same thing, "Who says men can't have profound, personal conversations?" That seems to sum up how the majority of men communicate; a few words, a lot of meaning.

A hospice patient once told me about his dad. He said as a little boy growing up his family would have large family picnics. He'd ask his Dad if he could go down to the creek with the other kids. His dad would say yes, adding, "If you come back crying, you better be bleeding." He knew that reply gave him the freedom to explore but he knew if anybody teased him he had to defend himself. The patient told me his dad was a man of few words but he was always teaching and guiding. Nurturing was Mom's department.

If your dad is here on Earth, make sure you tell him how proud you are of him and that he did a good job.

~ THANKSGIVING ~

THE WORD "THANKSGIVING" is obviously made of two words, "thanks" and "giving." "Thanks" is an expression of gratitude but "giving" is an action of gratitude. Giving doesn't necessarily mean giving something tangible such as money. It may be as simple as giving encouragement, giving someone your full attention, or most importantly, giving someone your time. Regardless, giving involves getting out of yourself. Although it may seem that saying thanks is enough, people may not believe what you say, they will believe what you do.

Hospice volunteers are a good example of demonstrating that giving thanks is an action, not just a word. Some volunteers want to give thanks to hospice because they experienced the comfort of end-of-life care with a family member through hospice, while some want to volunteer in order to give thanks to God for their blessings.

One of the many benefits of hospice care is that it allows family and friends to actively give thanks to someone in their life. Hospice allows grown children the honor of actively giving thanks to their mom or dad. We show them how to care for their parent in their last days, much like the parent cared for them in their first days. Having the opportunity to give thanks at the end of life is truly the best time to do it.

Thanksgiving is the holiday in which we give thanks to God for our blessings. As a suggestion for Thanksgiving, why not give thanks to God through acts of kindness and mercy, and not just say thanks?

~ VOLUNTEERS ARE NECESSARY ~

THE POWER OF volunteerism is astounding. It was through the drive and dedication of volunteers that the hospice movement evolved in earnest during the late 1960's in England. The first hospice in America was started in New Haven, Connecticut in 1974 by volunteers, and the fourth hospice in Ohio, where I volunteer, was started during 1984 in Lancaster, Ohio by volunteers.

According to Medicare's Conditions of Participation, volunteers must provide day-to-day administrative and/or direct patient care services in an amount that equals 5% of the total patient care hours of all paid hospice employees and contract staff. As hospice continues to grow, that mandate requires a steadily increasing number of hours to be provided by volunteers. I am proud to say that my hospice always exceeds the Medicare requirement.

Hospice volunteers are regular people who have unique personalities and skills. They are residents of this area who are sensitive to the needs of families and they are people who serve without financial compensation. To become a hospice volunteer, my hospice requires 22 hours of training. Topics covered in training deal with: family dynamics, the hospice philosophy, patient rights, stress management, disease process, death awareness, confidentiality, and boundary setting.

Within my hospice there are two areas of volunteerism available: patient contact and non-patient contact. The two groups are equal in their importance to hospice and to our patients.

Our non-patient contact volunteers work in many capacities such as filing, office receptionist and fundraising. I used to naively think that the non-patient contact volunteers were not affected by the emotional intensity of the patient-side hospice work. I was wrong. I was in the hospice office recently when I heard one of our office volunteers say to herself, "May God bless and welcome this person." She was removing a patient's folder from the "Active File" and moving it to the "Deceased File." That simple act of removing the paperwork meant that a person has now left this life. The volunteer's short, whispered prayer reminded me of how important all hospice volunteers are, and how they are blessed by the duties that they perform.

The varied interests and special talents of our volunteers greatly expand the number and scope of services hospice is able to offer. This alone enhances the patient and family quality of life. Some hospices offer massage therapy, music therapy, touch therapy, and children's grief programs. I heard of many examples demonstrating that volunteers always seem to be looking for ways to help. One male volunteer noticed the deer around the hospice home and worked to have a salt lick put on the grounds in an area that would be visible from many of the patient rooms. He also noticed how families and patients liked to watch the activity at the bird feeder in the front of the hospice home. He suggested, then installed, a bird feeder positioned outside each of the 12 patient rooms so that a patient could watch the birds while lying in bed. What an incredibly simple, yet profound idea that turned out to be. Watching the bird feeder benefits the person on service, their family, and our staff.

Through the commitment of being a hospice volunteer, volunteers act as a liaison between the hospice program and the community. They bring awareness of hospice's services and encourage support of hospice care within their circle of friends and family.

Volunteers also serve on our not-for-profit advisory board, assist at various hospice-sponsored functions, participate in health fairs and county fairs, and help with fundraising events.

The patient contact volunteers are in a position to receive privileges when working with a patient. They are given the privilege of entering into someone's life and helping them celebrate their personal history, their successes, and regrets. Patient contact volunteers may also be in the position to help a patient complete some final goals in life, such as a train layout for a grandson. And they may also be there when the patient experiences a "last." Life has as many "lasts" as it does "firsts," such as the last time a patient was able to lift a spoon or get out of bed without help.

Bereavement volunteers contact family and loved ones following the death of a patient. In many hospices volunteers make follow up phone calls and send cards to those who had a loved one on service. Bereavement volunteers offer support and compassion. Volunteers may make phone calls, do in-person visits, and help organize or co-facilitate support groups, all with the guidance of a grief coordinator. One of the many compassionate gestures the bereavement volunteers do is to call the survivor left alone, after a death, on an important date or anniversary. So many people are brought to tears when they tell me how important it was to know that their loved one had not been forgotten.

Many volunteer activities available in hospice don't involve direct contact with patients, yet all volunteers are blessed by what hospice does and hospice is definitely blessed by what its volunteers do. The Medicare requirement of having volunteers is one of the reasons that hospice is completely different than anything you have experienced in the medical field. They selflessly bring light and life to a person during the last stage of life.

~ What Needs Doing ~

I WAS TALKING to a friend of mine who mentioned that she was thinking about becoming a hospice patient care volunteer. She was hesitant because she didn't know what it entailed. Well, it's difficult to itemize what our patient care volunteers do, but I happened to have a copy of a poem by a hospice volunteer from Wisconsin. Regretfully, the person who gave the poem to me didn't know the author's name. The poem succinctly describes what hospice volunteers do. It follows:

"But what will you do? I don't know.

I'll have to see what needs doing.

Maybe I'll wash the dishes, or tell you a joke, or bring you some soup,

or play some cards. If you want to talk, I can listen.

If you don't want to talk, maybe I can answer the telephone.

If you're not sure you're doing what's best,

maybe I can tell you you're doing what's best,

maybe I can tell you you're doing just fine.

If you have to get some rest,

maybe you'll trust me to sit by their bed.

If you're angry, maybe I can say that's OK.

If your strength is failing, maybe I can reach out my hand

and keep you going. If you're falling apart, maybe I can put my arms around you

and hold you together. If you're feeling helpless, maybe we can pray together.

I'll have to see what needs doing. Maybe you won't need me for anything!

Maybe I'll just call or stop in to remind you

I'm standing by, ready to help if you do need me. "

That sums it up – in hospice, our volunteers just do what needs doing.

~ WHAT IS IT LIKE TO BE A HOSPICE PATIENT-CONTACT VOLUNTEER? ~

THERE ARE MANY areas of hospice in which to volunteer but the area that seems to generate the most apprehension, or fear, to someone considering volunteering for a hospice organization is that of patient-contact volunteer. I know that I was nervous about being involved with patient care, but at the same time I knew that it was something that I had to do. The primary purpose of the hospice patient-contact volunteer is to offer respite, or a rest, to the caregiver. Generally, the volunteer will stay with the patient while the caregiver runs errands, attends functions, or just takes a nap.

I've been a volunteer for over 20 years. It has been, and still is, a great experience for me. With a few patients, I was involved for a year or more and some of the patients I never met because plans changed. I quickly learned that there is no routine at the end of life. In the situations where I never met the patient it might have been that more family was able to help, maybe the patient moved in with a family caregiver, and sometimes the patient died before I made my first visit. Regardless of the circumstances, the volunteer always has the option to decline an assignment. No volunteer in hospice has to do something if they don't feel comfortable in a particular situation.

Not all of any hospices' patients are bedridden. Some of my patients were able to greet me at the door and some would be in a recliner in the living room when I came to visit. And every year we have a person on service ride with us in the Fourth of July Parade. The Christmas Parade has not cooperated weather wise to allow a person on service to be in it.

One of the prevalent myths is that hospice is a place. The thought is that when you sign on to hospice you have to go to their facility. With some hospices you do and with others you don't. At the hospice where I volunteer we take care of people where they live, whether it's at home, in a nursing home, an assisted living facility, or an apartment. When the patient lives at home, we give them the choice of what room to live in. In any case, hospice is focused on what the patient wants. I've had patients in nice neighborhoods and not so nice ones. In old homes, beautiful homes out in the country with a weeping willow by a pond, nursing homes and assisted living facilities, run down farm houses, apartments, and one patient in a camper in his backyard.

Just to give you an idea of what being a patient-care volunteer may involve I'll give a brief scenario, based only on personal experience, of the complete start to finish of a volunteer's involvement with a family:

I'll get a call from the hospice volunteer coordinator. I'll be asked if I'm ready for a new patient. I'll be given the particulars about the person's age, disease, who's the primary caregiver (PCG), where the person lives, and a brief description of the family dynamics. I say, "Yes, I'll accept them." (It is my choice to say yes or no). I am then given their personal contact information and then I'm "off to the races." I immediately call the PCG and try to set up a 5-minute meeting in their home so that I may introduce myself, find out their expectations and to set up a visiting schedule.

When the patient to whom I've been assigned lives at home, the most apprehensive part of the whole experience is walking up to the residence for the first time. There are so many unknowns as to what everyone looks like (particularly the patient), the appearance of the inside of the house, if there are pets (I keep doggy treats and cat treats in my truck), and if there are any "medical" smells in the house.

I also wonder about the anxiety level of the primary caregiver, and what room the patient is in. I've had patients with their hospital bed set up in bedrooms, living rooms, recreation rooms, unfinished basements, in the garage with their street rod, in their wood shop, and in the kitchen.

During the first visit, I try to evaluate who needs the most attention. Often, it's the primary caregiver. Generally during a visit, I spend time talking (re: listening) to the primary caregiver, who is generally the spouse, child, or parent. They are at their wits' end because of the end-of-life crisis of their loved one, while the patient is often at peace with their situation. The volunteer is the only person on the hospice staff who doesn't have an agenda or a specific purpose. Therefore, the volunteer is non-threatening and more able to help the family in whatever capacity they request. The scheduled visits continue for as long as the patient is on service. My involvement with a patient has lasted from as short as one visit to as long as 15 months. (A patient may stay on hospice service as long as they remain hospice appropriate.)

It is extremely important to understand that the end stage of any disease may leave the patient thin and gaunt. This isn't a beauty contest. The sole purpose of the volunteer is to give the people involved love and attention. The family member's appearance, housekeeping habits, and anything else are just not important.

I am usually notified by the hospice office of the patient's passing very soon after the event. A few times, I've been present as the patient died and in each instance the death was expected. The dying process is generally very slow. Yes, those were emotional and very spiritual events. I consider it an honor to have been there. However, many times the dying person wants to die alone and will wait until they are alone to die.

I always attend either the Calling Hours or the funeral service. There are usually photos on display or videos playing of the deceased, chronicling their life. It helps to look at the pictures because it helps to put everything into perspective and to see the patient as everyone else knew them. It's also important to the family for the volunteer to attend the service so that they can say thank you. At one of the calling hours, I was standing with my hands to my side. The deceased's wife came up to me and held each of my hands, still to my side, looked up at me and whispered, "Thank You." I broke down and cried. Crying is a part of being involved with patients and their families. It shows that the people of hospice do care and do have feelings for the patient and family.

Something that technology can't change is that life begins with family and ends with family. Through compassionate care provided by hospice staff, and its volunteers, the end of life can be a return to personal family time, a time before the modern age turned dying into a medical event. Through ordinary, everyday people hospice gives extraordinary care.

~ Endings to Beginnings ~

THE FIRST HOLIDAY of the holiday "trifecta," Thanksgiving, focuses on gratitude while the second, Christmas, focuses on love. The third holiday is New Year's Day. And the focus of New Year's is transition, from endings to beginnings.

During the week between Christmas and New Year's there are radio and TV shows that recount the year's biggest news stories, top songs, most popular movies, etc. And during this time there is also introspection about problems that we had during the past year and how to correct them. Many of us make our resolutions about how we are going to improve our lives. In order to make New Year's resolutions you must review your life. Taking time to review your life can actually be refreshing and may lift your spirits. It confirms that your life has meaning.

This year, instead of thinking only of correcting bad habits, consider thinking a little deeper.

Being with people in their last stage of life as they look back and review their life has taught me to do the same. One of the many benefits of hospice, especially the one where I volunteer, is that we offer a time of calm that allows the person to reflect upon their life.

People whom I got to know in their last stage of life have asked me, "what was your legacy last year and how will you be remembered when this year ends?" My conversations with them have brought me to internalize and think more seriously about how to live my life. Should there be any endings and possibly a beginning or two?

It's not too late to make some adjustments in your way of living for your life ahead. Begin the process of living in the manner which will create the legacy that you want leave.

~ WITHOUT CHARGING A PENNY ~

NOT LONG AFTER the hospice house where I volunteer opened I was standing on its front porch talking to a man who, to my surprise, told me that he was staying there for a five-day respite. During our conversation "Chuck" (not his real name) told me that he "...sure didn't deserve this." I assured him that he does.

He'd lived mostly in apartments and sleeping rooms for the last few months before he moved to the V.A. Center in Chillicothe, Ohio. Although still appearing somewhat healthy, he didn't have a long-life expectancy.

We talked a little about the progression of his illness. Then casually looking up at the hospice house's portico, he seemed to talk to himself saying, "Man, I don't deserve this. I've never experienced this amount of attention and great care."

Our conversation had started a little while earlier when he wanted to know what the catch was, as he politely added, "With no baloney." The catch being how can we provide the high level of service and give the amount of time we do to each patient without charging a penny?

By asking that question Chuck was inquiring about one of the many indiscernible things that hospice does to bring comfort and peace into a family's life. Most likely, a life that had been filled with stress, fear, and suffering. So, with no baloney, I'd like to explain how hospice does what it does without charging the recipient.

One of the subtle ways that we help our patients and their families to be at peace is not to charge them for our services. What? Many hospices, including mine, do not charge the family for our services. As Chuck asked me, "If you don't charge for your services then how do you pay your employees? And how do you maintain this wonderful hospice house?"

The answer is simple. We have several sources of income including a per diem (meaning "per day") payment from Medicare for each day that a patient is on our service. We also receive funds from the patient's insurance (we pay the deductible,) and, if the patient qualifies, we receive funds from Medicaid.

Even though we receive reimbursement for our basic services as all hospices do, there is still a very real need for additional funding. For example, most of our bereavement service costs are uncompensated. And we do not charge for our palliative care service expenses so they are absorbed by my hospice. Therefore, we do need financial help so that we can do all the little extras that no other hospice does.

We receive those additional funds through the generosity of companies and individuals, as well as grants from philanthropic foundations. Most smaller town hospices also benefit from various community groups. Such groups as car clubs, motorcycle clubs, hospital twigs, sororities, etc., may hold events to raise money for the local hospice. One younger couple who come to mind have been holding a motorcycle poker run annually since 2006. When it is finished, all my hospice has to do is send a representative to bring back the money.

My opinion is that hospice is by far the best thing that could happen during the worst time, short of a miracle cure. And we do it without charging a penny.

~ WHY VOLUNTEER? ~

I RECENTLY RECEIVED a letter from Dianne, a new hospice volunteer, which I feel nicely answers the question, "Why would you want to do *that*?!" She writes:

"Our youngest is now twenty-four and I am now able to spend some time giving back to our community. The more I learn about hospice the more I love it. We are truly one big family (at hospice) and I am proud to be a part of it.

"When I was nine years old I found an injured bird in our yard, so I fixed up a shoe box to make him comfortable and tried to take care of him. After a few days, the bird died. I was so sad. My mother assured me it was all okay because that birdie was with someone who cared for him during the last days of his life and he didn't die alone. Now that I volunteer with hospice I know what mother meant!"

"Hospice helps complete the cycle of life, whether we live a few days, a few years, or a hundred years. Someone is there to comfort you, guide you, care for you, and assist you through the end of human life as we know it here on Earth. With hospice, there is someone to walk you into the next life where we spend spiritually in eternity. I like that very much. It gives me great comfort to deal with the end of life in a normal, loving, and dignified manner."

I have been a volunteer with Diane for quite a few years. She is not only involved with patient contact, she also is very actively involved in fundraising. Part of what she does for us is to sew and make quilts to give to our patients. She demonstrates that a good reason to volunteer is to use your talents to help others.

~ Just A Simple Pinning ~

WHEN A PERSON signs on to the hospice where I volunteer, our social worker will sit down with the patient and their family and take the time to get to know them. Our care is holistic, meaning that it includes all aspects of a patient's life: physical, emotional, and spiritual. From what we learn, we can develop a plan of care based on how the patient would like to live.

The social worker will also ask about any hopes, wishes, or disappointments. We do this so that we can help them, if needed, complete any unfinished business. We might also learn what the patient considers to be an accomplishment and to learn of areas of satisfaction the patient had during his or her life.

If the patient, or family, mentions that the person was a military veteran, we will ask if they'd like to talk about it. Sometimes they do and sometimes they don't. If they do we will talk to them about their experiences, where they served, etc. We then ask if they would like to be thanked for their service through a military pinning service. I think in every case the answer has been, "Yes."

It's a simple pinning service that is conducted where the veteran lives, be it a facility or their home. For the pinning service, as many people as the veteran or their family want to attend may. Sometimes there are many in attendance and sometimes just a few. It has never seemed to matter how many were there.

I spoke to a group several months ago, and a woman told me that we did the service for her dad at her house where she was caring for him. Only she, her dad, our social worker and one of our patient care volunteers, himself a veteran, were there in the man's bedroom.

It was late in the evening but indications were that he might not have too much longer to live so now was the time. The volunteer read the proclamation thanking him for his service, pinned him on his pajamas' lapel and presented him with a Certificate of Appreciation. He then took a step back and saluted the patient. The patient had seemed to be in a deep sleep but when our volunteer saluted him, he lifted his right hand, with fingers straight, as far as he could in order to return the salute. The daughter started to cry as she told the story and to be honest, so did I. This little ceremony is so simple, yet so profound.

During the week that contains Veteran's Day, my hospice always makes arrangements to conduct the same pinning service at most of the area nursing or assisted living facilities that have veterans as residents. I have been privileged to attend several of these events. One pinning service, in particular, occurred last year at an assisted living facility. There were 7 or 8 veterans present. Most were in wheelchairs but two insisted on standing, much to the chagrin of the facilities' staff.

The attending hospice volunteer, himself a veteran, read the proclamation. He pinned each man who was at attention, whether sitting or standing, with eyes straight ahead. All of them had family present. Afterward, one of the veterans came over to tell me how important the ceremony was to him. He said that it was the first time that he was honored since being discharged after serving in Korea. The "Forgotten War" he called it.

"I've been to parades and heard speeches and read articles in the paper, but this was the first time in 62 years that someone ever shook my hand, gave me a certificate of appreciation, and said 'Thank you' directly to me."

At first, he told me that the lack of acknowledging his military service didn't bother him because he hasn't been on the front. He had been in an artillery unit (yes, he was hard of hearing) but eventually was given a new assignment. He said that in Korea nobody was really safe, but "I was back a-ways and felt pretty safe."

I asked him what his new duty was after he left his artillery unit. He said, "They moved me to where the action was." He turned, looked outside for a minute, took a deep breath and said, "My job was to make sure the correct dog tag was on each body before we'd load them on the plane. I'd open the body bag, check each one, say a short prayer, then zip the bag closed and place them on a pallet. Then I'd go to the next one. When I was all done, I'd get on a lift truck and lift up the pallet, place it in a C-47 (military plane). Then me and the plane crew would salute the dead."

Then he told me, "You know, I hate to say this but it was so nice to see someone who was just shot. So many times, I'd open the bag and there were just pieces." He was quiet for a few seconds, "I still see 'em. The worst ones were killed by a bayonet or a shell. It was hard to identify them. When I'd open a body bag, sometimes I didn't know what part of the body I was looking at. After a few of these, it was a relief to identify someone who was only shot. War makes you that way." He said that it wasn't a job that he got thanked for too much. But he knew it was important nonetheless.

Again, he thanked my hospice for giving him the recognition and said, "I always thought sending the dead back home was the most important thing I ever did."

And it was just a simple pinning service. Thank a veteran.

~ Darling, We Made It ~

THE MAN HAD been on hospice service for several months. He and his wife were quietly anticipating their wedding anniversary but recently his illness wasn't cooperating. In the early part of the week his health began to decline and it was decided to bring him into the hospice facility to give him some extra attention. His hospice nurse knew how important this anniversary was to the couple and it was hoped that the extra attention afforded at the facility would enable him to live to celebrate his anniversary with his lifelong friend and companion.

The man had always been adamant that he wanted to die at home, although in this situation conventional wisdom dictated that he go to the facility. Hopefully, he would stay for just a few days until he stabilized, then return home.

On Thursday, it looked like he might not make it. Their 58th wedding anniversary was on Sunday. The facility Kitchen Manager, Linda, was baking a gorgeous wedding anniversary cake, figuring that they would celebrate the anniversary there.

The patient was declining and it looked like his Hour may be approaching. He would probably die there. Yet, his wife knew that he wanted to be in the warmth and familiarity of his own home. Our patient's desires always come first, so on Saturday afternoon it was decided that he would be transported home to fulfill his wish.

Linda finished the anniversary cake about an hour after the patient was taken home. As luck would have it one of our volunteers, Chris, stopped by the facility to visit another patient. The cook mentioned her dilemma of having the anniversary cake but no way to deliver it. Chris agreed to take it, commenting that it was a coincidence that it was his anniversary on Sunday, as well.

Chris gingerly put the cake in his car and left to make the all-important delivery. After he was gone, Linda decided to bake a cake for Chris and his bride of over 30 years. She knew that two couples were being blessed on this anniversary.

As Chris was driving over on his cake-mission-of-mercy he got to thinking of all of the wonderful things that he had been involved with as a volunteer. So many things that seemed insignificant at the time but were overwhelmingly important to the recipient. All were spur of the moment occurrences. And very few of these situations were covered in his volunteer training. In fact, delivering anniversary cakes wasn't even mentioned. He smiled.

It was early evening when Chris pulled into the driveway. Luckily the cake was still in one piece. The couple's daughter met Chris when he got out of his car. Placing her hand on his arm she softly said, "Dad's not doing very well."

"How about if I bring the cake in and let your Mom admire it." It was obviously not the time to have cake, but he didn't know what else to say. Anyone who has entered a home when someone is preparing to cross to the Other Side is keenly aware of the spiritually charged atmosphere. Time stands still; there is only sacred silence. The family was holding a vigil in the bedroom and his wife was sitting at his bedside. Chris stayed a few minutes, then left.

Just before midnight, the wife quietly went to the kitchen, cut a small piece of cake, placed it on a plate and returned to her love's bedside. In the room, there were a few sniffles. The only movement was someone occasionally wiping a tear. With the wall clock tolling midnight, his wife scooped a bit of icing on her finger and slowly, tenderly wiped just a little on his lip. "Happy Anniversary, darling, we made it," she whispered, then gently kissed him.

With a faint smile, he looked at her, looked up, and was gone.

The couple celebrated their anniversary, their way... on their anniversary day. That is what hospice does.

~ LAUGHING MATTERS ~

THERE ARE A lot of articles written about the hospice philosophy, hospice care, who is eligible for hospice care, etc. But not many articles are written about humor, or laughter, in the hospice setting. Having been a hospice patient care volunteer for over 20 years and a paid employee for over 11 years, I know that hospice is serious business. I also know that hospice, especially the one where I volunteer, celebrates life. And life may involve laughter, but hospice is no laughing matter, is it?

Of course, we've all heard the overworked phrase, "Laughter is the best medicine." It may be an overworked phrase, but it's also a well-documented truth. Laughter is just as necessary in life as are tears. A friend of mine told me that laughter may be the best medicine, but if you are really sick, maybe you should call a doctor. Good advice.

It is important to know that used correctly, humor does not disrespect the situation nor diminish its gravity. It can allow what is happening to begin to be discussed. Humor may open the door to acceptance and healing. It's up to those involved to find the humor is any given situation.

Humor may be in the form of a funny situation or a joke. In my case I can never remember a joke so years ago I began writing them down after I heard one that I liked. I've kept those jokes in a binder. After I get to know a patient and it seems like the right thing to do (sometimes it's not), I will bring that binder with me when I visit them. I'll ask the patient and family if they'd mind if I read from my binder. It has never failed that when I bring the joke binder we all have a great time. They invariably tell me that they haven't had a good laugh like that in quite a while.

There was a particular family I visited as a patient care volunteer who requested what they called, a "groaner-type" joke when I arrived for my weekly visit. A groaner-type joke would be for example, "Why did the cowboy buy a Dachshund?" Answer, "Because he wanted to get a 'long little doggy'" (groan).

When I would arrive to visit, his wife would answer the door and ask," Do you know any groaners?" I would answer, "Yes. Did you hear about the man who was reading a book on antigravity? He just couldn't put it down." She'd laugh and ask me, "Did you hear about the Siamese twins who moved to England...so the other one could drive?" Then we'd go back to the patient's room and he couldn't wait to hear the jokes. He'd always have one ready. For example, "Did you know that trying to write with a broken pencil is pointless? The whole situation was fun to me. I remember thinking that I never thought that I would have so much fun visiting a patient.

Exchanging bad jokes was fun and it made the patient, his wife, and I think of a silly joke before my weekly visit. There is no doubt that he and his wife were having fun too. Yes, the patient and spouse knew he was terminally ill but we had fun in spite of it.

One of my hospice chaplains, Karl, tells the story of a terminally ill patient who is lying in his bed at home and smells the aroma of cookies wafting through the house.

"Honey," he calls out, "Those cookies smell so good, may I have one?"

"Certainly not," she replies, "Those are for your wake!"

In one study of humor in the hospice setting it was determined that humor helped to maintain a sense of belonging. It helped patients to relax. It offered a feeling of warmth, lightheartedness, and delight. Humor was a life-enricher and a life enhancer.

A study done on nurse-based home visits found that humor was present in 85% of 132 observed home hospice visits. Of these visits, hospice patients initiated humor 70% of the time. In this study, and others as well, humor was spontaneous and frequent.

A while back, I was accompanying one of my hospice's nurses while she visited a patient in their home. The family pet was a cockatiel (a bird similar to a parrot). The family would leave the bird cage door open so that the bird could get out and stretch if it wanted to. While our nurse was sitting next to the patient the bird flew over and landed on the nurse's shoulder. Without hesitation, the nurse put her hand over her eye and said, "Aye, matey." as if she were a pirate. Everyone had a good laugh.

Instances of humorous interactions between hospice personnel and patients can be a prevalent part of everyday care giving work. According to the researcher in the study mentioned above, "Our research suggests that nurses and other healthcare professionals don't need to suppress humor. They should trust their instincts about when it's appropriate."

Humor shows the human side of hospice's staff. It's also an important aspect of communication. Patients will observe the nurse or aide for a response to humor. An open, accepting response to humor signals understanding, while a negative or no response may serve to isolate the patient.

The hospice where I volunteer helps people to celebrate life. One way to celebrate life is to enjoy the moment, regardless of the circumstance. Laughter is a very effective way to do that. I'm often asked, "How can you work in hospice? Isn't it sad?" It's hard to believe that not only is it very rewarding to volunteer with hospice, but sometimes it can also be fun. Yes, laughing matters.

~ LIFE'S TWO BIG EVENTS ~

HOSPICE EVOLVED IN the late 1960's. Personally, a lot has happened since then. For example, for me in the late 1960's it was long hair then; now it's no hair. Back then the police told me to slow down; now my doctor tells me to slow down.

Society's way of approaching life's two big events, birth and death, has also changed. In the late 1960's the Lamaze method of childbirth developed. This method allowed the father to be a part of the childbirth process. When I was young, the method of birthing was the mother went to the Delivery Room, the father went to the Waiting Room, and soon the baby appeared. And, according to old cartoons, at some point in history the baby was brought by a stork.

Also in the late 1960's, a philosophy developed that dealt with the opposite end of the spectrum, i.e., death. That philosophy became known as "hospice" and was, in part, the result of the research by Dr. Elisabeth Kubler-Ross. She authored a book entitled, "*On Death and Dying*" that became the impetus to medically confront end-of-life issues. Up to that point, as someone entered the last stage of life, they were sequestered in a "Rest Home" or facility of some sort and often not told of their condition so that they wouldn't get upset.

Society has definitely improved its handling of life's greatest events. Life begins with family and ends with family. Hospice is there to help and support your family through life's second big event.

~ Put Your Life Back in Order ~

I WAS TALKING TO a hospice nurse practitioner and she mentioned how often she hears the comment, "If only I knew what hospice did, I would have called sooner." It's very hard to describe exactly what we do because each patient and family situation is unique. But probably the number one item we provide for someone dealing with a very serious medical crisis is to put everyone's life back in order.

In a typical situation, up until a family calls hospice, there have been innumerable trips to medical offices and facilities. Most likely there have been many doctors and a variety of specialists who all have something to do with caring for the patient. And occasionally not all of these medical personnel are on the same page. Sometimes information is not shared. Being under stress and new to all of this, sometimes the family just wonders what is going on.

When hospice comes into a family's life due to a member being terminally ill, their lives improve immensely. We put order into what was chaos. We are experts in our line of work and we often answer many questions that people didn't know they had.

It's important to know that hospice does not sign anyone on to service until it's certain that the patient has exhausted all standard care options. For a family, that is the hardest part to accept. But once accepted, hospice can put your life back in order.

~ She Did it Again ~

IT SEEMS THAT during the oddest of times, a hospice employee might hear a wonderful story of the effecy they have on people. At the end of an emotionally draining day, one of our hospice social workers, Ellen, was standing in line at her bank. A woman came over and asked if that was Brinkli who was with her. Brinkli must have recognized the woman because she moved around to join in the conversation. Ellen acknowledge that, indeed, she was Brinkli.

The woman then began to tell Ellen in great detail how wonderful and attentive Brinkli was to her family while her mother was staying a few days at our hospice's facility. The woman got her phone out and showed Ellen her screen-saver. It was a photo of her husband sitting at her mother's bedside cupping Brinkli's head in his hands. The woman said that he was telling Brinkli how he felt and thanking her for being there.

Sometimes in stressful situations it's the one without an agenda who seems to be most effective in comforting. It's often the one who just enters the room to be with the patient, and to just listen if the patient wants to talk, who seems to be the most comforting to the patient or their family.

Leaving the bank, Ellen realized that she no longer felt the stress of her day since the woman took the time to thank her for Brinkli. Oh, did I mention that Brinkli is one of our hospice's therapy dogs? Sounds like Brinkli did it again.

~ Still a Salesman ~

ABOUT FIVE YEARS into my career as a volunteer at the local hospice I was assigned a patient in a nursing home. When my hospice assigns a patient to a volunteer, the volunteer always has the right to say no. The Volunteer Coordinator will call and ask if the volunteer is willing to accept a new patient. If the answer is yes then the Volunteer Coordinator gives the volunteer basic information about the patient's illness, family dynamics, where the patient lives, etc. She will also supply any pertinent information as to the person's likes, hobbies, background, etc. If the volunteer is amicable to the offer then they will accept the patient. There is never any pressure for a volunteer to accept an assignment.

In this particular case, the man that I agreed to visit had been living in this nursing home for over eight years. He was described as being noncommutative. He signed on to our service due to heart disease and he also had a secondary diagnosis of early stages of dementia. Even though it seemed like this could be one of my quiet, uneventful assignments, my experience taught me that sometimes the patients who turn out to be the most interesting patients may not sound so interesting on paper. His name was "Hank" and, according to the information that I was given, he had various sales jobs during his career.

My way of getting to know a new person is to make an initial visit with no plans or expectations. Sometimes a person's mental or physical status may change from when I was given their information to when I meet them face to face, so I always meet the person before I decide on a plan of action.

During my first visit, it wasn't long before we were in a conversation. He was described as noncommutative, but in reality all he needed was someone to take the time to be with him. As I was leaving I told him the day and time that I was coming to visit him again. When I arrived on the day of my next visit, the nurse on his floor greeted me by name because Hank had been asking all day if it was time for me to visit yet. He may have had early stages of dementia but he was still alive and he had purpose; to wait for a visitor.

I learned during my first visit that the patient had been a car salesman early in his career. As luck would have it I collected automobilia. i.e.; items related to automobiles. In my collection were two large scrap books that contained car ads that had been cut out of *Life* and *Look* magazines from the 1950's, the same era that Hank was selling cars.

For the next visit, I brought in those two scrapbooks much to the delight of Hank. He evidently sold less popular brands of cars such as Studebaker, Nash and other long forgotten makes because he'd thumb right past the Ford, Chevrolet and Chrysler ads and stop at an ad for a lesser known brand.

He was excited to see a Nash advertisement. He pointed out the features of it from the ad's picture and told about the size engine, color options, and how comfortable the ride was. In fact, the next two visits were spent with the two of us laughing and talking about cars and how much better the cars used to be.

As this visit came to an end, he offered to go with me to the front door to see me off. I helped him into his wheelchair, put the foot rests down, the brake levers up, and we were ready to go. He was still in his salesman state of mind from looking at the automobile ads because as we were preparing to move Hank showed me the features of his wheelchair. He pointed out the chrome finish, the dark blue padded seat, and individual brakes levers for each wheel. Yes, this model had a brake lever for each wheel.

He started to move forward but quickly tired so I pushed him down the hall at a leisurely pace and we eventually arrived at the front door. After we said our goodbyes he looked at me with a sheepish look on his face. Then it hit me; if he was too tired or weak to move himself in the wheelchair to the door, he is certainly not able to do it on the return trip to his room.

Did I mention that Hank's nursing home was a sprawling facility and he was living in the back end, in the last room of a long hall? Basically, he was as far away from the front door as possible. Obviously, this should have occurred to me when our little adventure began, but he was being so friendly and polite that I didn't want to offend him by turning down such a generous offer. So instead of me being escorted to the door by my patient, I pushed him to the front door.

We said our goodbyes and then I pushed him back to his room. Once I had him settled back in bed I walked all the way back to the front door and left. (Thus completing my exercise requirements for the day, I might add.) As I approached the front door for that second time I remember smiling and thinking to myself, "Hank was so enthusiastic about those old car ads that I think he could have sold me a Nash."

Until hospice had been called, the patient spent most of his time lethargically in bed. His heart condition had weakened him and the beginnings of dementia caused him to occasionally be confused. In the last stage of life the weakening of the body and mind are the hardest realities to accept. The hospice where I volunteer helps people on its service to focus on what can still be done and encourages them to make living worthwhile.

Even at the end of his life, Hank awakened to what had been denied him for so long; he was still a salesman.

~ VOLUNTEER THERE? ~

ON A PLEASANT June afternoon one of the hospice volunteers, where I also volunteer, was spending time with "Ann," a woman seemingly much too young to be on our service. The volunteer had accepted the patient assignment several weeks earlier and got to know Ann fairly well. During that time, the volunteer learned that as her illness progressed Ann longed to be on the back of her husband's Harley cruising through the countryside. It didn't look like that was going to happen and she was despondent. Well, as it turned out the volunteer, who happens to have the perfect name for a hospice volunteer, Joy, also liked to ride. She decided to do something about the situation.

There are certain things that just shouldn't be done when someone is as ill as Ann, even on hospice care, but Joy was not deterred. As a volunteer for hospice, Joy knew that she had to use her imagination to somehow help Ann experience one more ride. Joy put her hand in Ann's and said, "Between you and me, I think we can do something about being on a Harley." Joy helped her lay back, told her to close her eye s and get set for a ride.

Joy told Ann that she was going to put her onto a motorcycle. After Joy made sure that Ann was comfortable she told her to get ready and hang on tight. As she talked, Ann felt the excitement while they "mounted up." The big Harley was pulsating and wanting to go. They slowly left the drive and Joy said that she was gradually lifting her feet up onto the pegs. Down the road they went. Because it was mid-June, Joy pointed out that the flowers were in full bloom, grass was intensely green and the tassels on the knee-high corn stalks were oh so fragrant. The deep rumble of the bike created a serenity that only a biker would understand. They leaned slightly to the left in a gradual turn and dip in the road, then to the right as the bike went up over a rise. It was just as Ann remembered it.

What started as a smile continued to grow until Ann was laughing. "This is great!" she exclaimed. For those few moments, the patient was riding on the back of her husband's bike. The sensations that she felt on that little excursion were the reasons she was holding on to life. She enjoyed the "trip" immensely. Once it was over, Ann slowly turned her head on the pillow and was fast asleep. Joy patted Ann's hand and left the room.

Left the room?! Yes, the patient and the volunteer had never left her room in The Pickering House, our hospice's in-patient facility. The "trip" began when the volunteer gently assisted the patient in lying back down in her bed to a position that did not cause discomfort. Joy asked Ann to close her eyes and "enjoy the ride" as she described a perfect ride in the country. Ann became so absorbed in Joy's description that I wouldn't doubt she checked to make sure that she didn't have any bugs in her teeth when it was over.

Our patient contact volunteer had given someone what she had been longing for four so long. What fighting a disease had taken from her life was given back by a non-medical volunteer who understood what was deep down important at this time in life. That is what hospice volunteers do; put purposeful life back into a person's life. And so many of the things that our patients are longing for at the end of life aren't necessarily a trip to the sea shore or Disney World. To someone not familiar with the emotional climate during the end of life, these inveterate longings of the terminally ill seem too mundane for anyone to normally think of. Many of the longings are of the one-last-time variety. Ann wanted to ride on a motorcycle one last time and her hospice volunteer used her creativity to accomplish it. Invariably the simplest requests from our patients seem to hold the greatest importance.

I think that one of the reasons so many people are surprised at the relief they feel when hospice becomes involved is because they didn't realize we focus on the human aspect of the end of life. We are interested in immediately giving the person on our service time to enjoy their life. We take the time to learn what is important to the ill person.

Because they take the time to listen, hospice volunteers bolster the ill person's self-respect. For so long during the progression of the illness, what the sick person wanted became secondary to what the treatment required. Now someone is not only listening to them but responding to what they want. They feel noticed and important again; what they want now matters to someone.

Besides giving an ill person their self-respect back, hospice can also give them purpose. Now they have someone who will listen and help them focus on attaining what they have been longing for, regardless of their condition. Disease be damned!

One of the people who visited my hospice's booth at the county fair told me that the volunteer who visited her sister helped them to put the "humanness" back into what was going on. As the person told me, "The volunteer thought of little things to do that we should've known to do. But since all the fuss over the disease had been going on for so long we just seemed to forget the simple things. Our volunteer helped us to get back into a comfortable routine of daily living. She was wonderful."

"Volunteer there? I don't think so," is a fairly common reply at the thought of volunteering at the local hospice. Numerous people have told me that they could never work with terminally ill people. Actually, they don't have to. There are two areas of volunteering: patient contact and non-patient involvement. In the non-patient arena, our volunteers help with fundraising, office work, and other various areas of patient support. Helping to plan and assist with fundraising events are always a lot of fun. There are also a few crafty volunteers who get together to help make blankets, quilts and anything else for patients that they can think of. Our volunteers are important and we listen to them.

Our census of people on service grows because more learn about the goodness of hospice. There is a continual need for a few more non-patient and patient contact volunteers. Volunteering at a hospice might be more enjoyable than you ever thought. Someone once told me the last good thing that happened to her mom was a hospice volunteer. That person could be you.

~ WHERE'D EVERYONE GO? ~

IT SEEMS LIKE when you leave the cemetery it's all over. Everyone goes home, the phone calls offering to help have ceased, and you are encouraged to focus on adjusting to your new life. But think about it – just because their heart stops beating doesn't mean that your heart stops loving.

In hospice, we know that after the numbness and shock wear off, after all the if-there's-anything-I-can-do-just-call-me statements have stopped, the real grief begins to develop. At this stage, the grieving family may be avoided because it's uncomfortable to be near them. There are so many awkward situations when an acquaintance is grieving.

Hospice is not about medicine. It's about you. Without the support of hospice, when the patient enters the last stage of life, all of the focus is on the illness. Very little effort is dedicated to the patient's or the family's emotional needs during their illness, except for maybe a free cup of coffee in the waiting room. And no thought is given to what happens after the patient dies. "Not my problem," seems to be the extent of it.

The purpose of hospice is to deal with the physical, emotional, and spiritual needs of the patient and family before the passing, and to maintain that effort with the family for over a year after the passing. There is no cost to the family for this.

Your local hospice knows that you alone must endure your grief, but you don't have to be alone. After your loved one dies, hospice will be there for a year of more if needed.

~ Why Not Tell Them Now ~

I RECEIVED AN invitation to my Aunt Ruth's 90th birthday party. "No presents, just your presence, please," it read. The only thing that my Aunt Ruth wanted for her birthday was for people to show up and enjoy themselves. She was always a great conversationalist and all she wanted for her birthday was to talk to family and friends. She got her wish.

My Aunt was a very proper woman who knew how things should be. She never corrected any of her nieces or nephews directly but would say, "I don't know about that," if we mentioned that we wanted to do something that she didn't approve of. Of all of my aunts, Aunt Ruth stood out among all the rest. And as I was soon to find out, all my cousins felt the same way.

I have to admit that I've been to a lot of birthday parties. This one was one of the best and by far the most memorable. It was held in the Community Center in the village of Greenhills. It's a suburb of Cincinnati that is completely surrounded by Winton Woods Park. Both the location and the weather were perfect.

In attendance were not only a nice percentage of her nieces and nephews, but also the people with whom she worked from years ago. I was surprised to see so many people she knew in her working life attending, since by this time Aunt Ruth had been retired for over 25 years. It was great for me to visit with so many of my cousins at one time on a happy occasion. So many times, I only get to see them during someone's Calling Hours. This was a nice, unhurried time to visit with everyone.

After the fellowship and dinner, it was about time to leave. My Aunt Ruth's only child, Patty, stood up and thanked everyone for coming to wish her mom a happy birthday. Then she mentioned that since there was such a wide variety of people present who knew her mom at different stages of her life, "Why don't we start at my right and just mention a favorite short story about Mom, a pleasant memory, or just simply how you knew her."

That simple little request turned into two hours of joy as people who worked with Aunt Ruth, neighbors from the old neighborhood and all of us cousins told short stories of my Aunt. One of my cousins mentioned how they weren't allowed in the Living Room because it was for "Company." Aunt Ruth didn't want that room torn up. We all roared with laughter, because each cousin could relate to that. Another cousin added how, when they would visit Aunt Ruth, their dad would pull over about a block away and remind them to stay out of the Living Room. Past office mates told how Aunt Ruth, as an accounting firm's office manager, was very strict and didn't let even the slightest error slide by. But she corrected an employee in such a way that it was almost like a compliment. The stories kept coming as at least sixty people told their own stories of Aunt Ruth.

We were so involved in what was going on that I don't think anyone realized that the Community Center staff had cleaned off the tables, put everything away and many had left for the evening. Only the manager stayed. We had overextended our welcome by quite a bit. As everyone left, we kept the conversation going in the parking lot. That event had stirred everyone's memories of growing up. It was a unifying event not only for my family but for everyone who knew Ruth Loftus. And I think it overwhelmed her daughter, Patty. She never expected that everyone would have something to say and that it would have such a positive effect on all present.

On the way home I started thinking, why do we wait until visiting hours to reminisce about someone's life? Why don't we do it while they can hear it and enjoy it like we did for Aunt Ruth? Maybe at the next birthday party you attend for someone in your family or a life-long friend, why not ask everyone to share a short story, a brief memory, or simply say how they met the person? It will be a joy to all present, especially the guest of honor and their family.

My Aunt was among the fortunate people who were able to hear nice things said about them by family and friends...while she could still hear them. Many nice things were said about my Dad and Mom at their respective funerals, but I wished that they could have heard them. Granted, it's nice for family members to hear nice things at the Calling Hours, but from my experience, it's much more fun to hear things at a party.

When the dying process starts, families will often gather at the bedside. For those fortunate enough to be at someone's bedside as their Hour approaches, there is an opportunity to tell the patient of happy memories the two of you share. This is important even if the person seems to be non-responsive. It is believed that hearing is the last of the five senses to leave.

In one particular situation, as a hospice volunteer, I received a call at work by my volunteer supervisor telling me that my patient was nearing the end. The dying process had started and there might be only hours remaining. I was told that the family requested that I be there in order to say good-bye to their Dad.

He was one of those patients where everything just clicked. We got along just fine. His wife had died several years earlier and he had spent several lonely years before he developed a terminal illness. He and I got along really well, we had many similar interests, and the same offbeat humor. I know full well when I meet a new patient that it will be generally only for a little while. But saying good-bye can be emotionally difficult, especially when a friendship develops.

This was the first time that I had been asked by a family to be at such an important event. I was humbled and afraid. What do I say? I was trying to think of something profound, something that the family would talk about for years to come. Nothing came to mind so I simply prayed for Divine guidance. The drive from work to the patient's bedside took about 45 minutes and during that time I prayed for wisdom and I prayed for the right words. The ride was a very quick 45 minutes and before I knew it, I was walking into his nursing home room.

His two daughters, both in their 40's, and their husbands were there, as well as several other family members. I don't think that I said anything profound, I just told him the truth. I told him what a good person he was. I recalled all the things we did since I've known him, and that because of all the love being shown to him during his illness, he must have done a lot of good for others during his life.

Weeks later, the hospice nurse told me how much my patient's two daughters appreciated the fact that I came to talk to their dad.

One of the nice things about telling someone how much they mean to you, especially during a birthday party or other gathering, is that it's a happy occasion. Someone always remembers a funny story about the person. I also noticed that as everyone shared stories about my aunt, no one mentioned anything about her possessions or her beautiful house. Well, except for maybe her Living Room that was saved for "company." For the most part, the stories were about her and her positive effect on people. She loved it and so did her daughter.

Senior citizens may avoid talking about the past so others won't regard them as senile. However, it's different in a crowd – it becomes a unifying event. At one time, bringing up old memories was considered living in the past. We now know that it is very therapeutic. I hope you think of this the next time you gather with friends or family. Reminiscing about someone will give them a lift and it will result in you feeling better, too. Why not tell them now before it's too late?

CPSIA information can be obtained
at www.ICGtesting.com
Printed in the USA
LVOW13*1221130418
573330LV00001B/2/P